Diabetic Cookbook For Two

4th edition
By Don Orwell

http://SuperfoodsToday.com

Your Free Gift

As a way of saying thanks for your purchase, I'm offering you my FREE eBook that is exclusive to my book and blog readers.

Superfoods Cookbook - Book Two has over 70 Superfoods recipes and complements Superfoods Cookbook Book One and it contains Superfoods Salads, Superfoods Smoothies and Superfoods Deserts with ultra-healthy non-refined ingredients. All ingredients are 100% Superfoods.

It also contains Superfoods Reference book which is organized by Superfoods (more than 60 of them, with the list of their benefits), Superfoods spices, all vitamins, minerals and antioxidants. Superfoods Reference Book lists Superfoods that can help with 12 diseases and 9 types of cancer.

http://www.SuperfoodsToday.com/FREE

Table of Contents

Superfoods Introduction

Superfoods are high in fiber, thermogenic, low in saturated fat, have tons of antioxidants, probiotic, vitamins, minerals, high in Omega 3 fats and above all tasty.

Superfoods Diabetic Diet works because it's return to the type of food your body naturally craves and was designed for. Whole foods Superfoods is the food humans consumed for literally millions of years. Superfoods are nutritionally dense foods that are widely available and which offer tremendous dietary and healing potential. Superfoods Diet is the only diet that doesn't restrict any major type of food. If features:

• Healthy Fats: Olive Oil, Nuts, Seeds, Coconut Oil, Avocado

• Proteins: Salmon, Beans, Organic Chicken, Grass-Fed Beef, Pork Tenderloin, Lentils

• Non-gluten Carbs: Certain Fruits (mostly berries), Leafy Vegetables, and small quantities of Oats, Brown Rice, Quinoa, Buckwheat

• Simple non-processed Dairy: Greek Yogurt, Farmer's Cheese, Goat Cheese

• Antioxidants: Garlic, Ginger, Turmeric, Cacao, Cinnamon, Berries

This book is suitable for diabetics with diabetes type 2.

Diabetic Cooking for One

Allergy labels: SF – Soy Free, GF – Gluten Free, DF – Dairy Free, EF – Egg Free, V - Vegan, NF – Nut Free

Condiments

Basil Pesto

- 1 cup basil
- 1/3 cup cashews
- 2 garlic cloves, chopped
- 1/2 cup olive oil or avocado oil

Process basil, cashews and garlic until smooth. Add oil in a slow stream. Process to combine. Transfer to a bowl. Season with salt and pepper. Stir to combine. Allergies: SF, GF, DF, EF, V

Cilantro Pesto

- 1 cup cilantro
- 1/3 cup cashews
- 2 garlic cloves, chopped
- 1/2 cup olive oil or avocado oil

Process cilantro, cashews and garlic. Add oil in a slow stream. Process to combine. Transfer to a bowl. Season with salt and pepper. Stir to combine. Allergies: SF, GF, DF, EF, V

Sundried Tomato Pesto

- 3/4 cup sundried tomatoes
- 1/3 cup cashews
- 2 garlic cloves, chopped
- 1/2 cup <u>olive</u> oil or <u>cumin</u> oil

Process tomato, cashews and garlic. Add oil in a slow stream. Process to combine. Transfer to a bowl. Season with salt and pepper. Stir to combine. Allergies: SF, GF, DF, EF, V

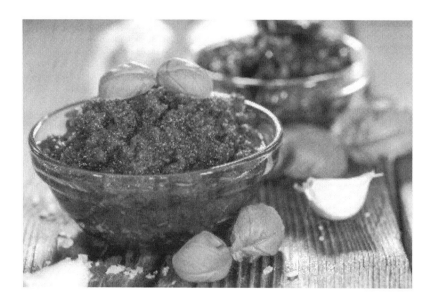

Broths

Some recipes require a cup or more of various broths, vegetable, beef or chicken broth. I usually cook the whole pot and freeze it.

Vegetable broth

Servings: 6 cups

Ingredients

- 1 tbsp. coconut oil
- 1 large onion
- 2 stalks celery, including some leaves
- 2 large carrots
- 1 bunch green onions, chopped
- 8 cloves garlic, minced
- 8 sprigs fresh parsley
- 6 sprigs fresh thyme
- 2 bay leaves
- 1 tsp. salt
- 2 quarts water

Instructions - Allergies: SF, GF, DF, EF, V, NF

Chop veggies into small chunks. Heat oil in a soup pot and add onion, scallions, celery, carrots, garlic, parsley, thyme, and bay leaves. Cook over high heat for 5 to 7 minutes, stirring occasionally.

Bring to a boil and add salt. Lower heat and simmer, uncovered, for 30 minutes. Strain. Other ingredients to consider: broccoli stalk, celery root

Chicken Broth

Ingredients

- 4 lbs. fresh chicken (wings, necks, backs, legs, bones)
- 2 peeled onions or 1 cup chopped leeks
- 2 celery stalks
- 1 carrot
- 8 black peppercorns
- 2 sprigs fresh thyme
- 2 sprigs fresh parsley
- 1 tsp. salt

Instructions - Allergies: SF, GF, DF, EF, NF

Put cold water in a stock pot and add chicken. Bring just to a boil. Skim any foam from the surface. Add other ingredients, return just to a boil, and reduce heat to a slow simmer. Simmer for 2 hours. Let cool to warm room temperature and strain. Keep chilled and use or freeze broth within a few days. Before using, defrost and boil.

Beef Broth

Ingredients

- 4-5 pounds beef bones and few veal bones
- 1 pound of stew meat (chuck or flank steak) cut into 2-inch chunks
- Olive oil
- 1-2 medium onions, peeled and quartered
- 1-2 large carrots, cut into 1-2 inch segments
- 1 celery rib, cut into 1 inch segments
- 2-3 cloves of garlic, unpeeled
- Handful of parsley, stems and leaves
- 1-2 bay leaves
- 10 peppercorns

Instructions - Allergies: SF, GF, DF, EF, NF

Heat oven to 375°F. Rub olive oil over the stew meat pieces, carrots, and onions. Place stew meat or beef scraps, stock bones, carrots and onions in a large roasting pan. Roast in oven for about 45 minutes, turning everything half-way through the cooking.

Place everything from the oven in a large stock pot. Pour some boiling water in the oven pan and scrape up all of the browned bits and pour all in the stock pot.

Add parsley, celery, garlic, bay leaves, and peppercorns to the pot. Fill the pot with cold water, to 1 inch over the top of the bones. Bring the stock pot to a regular simmer and then reduce the heat to low, so it just barely simmers. Cover the pot loosely and let simmer low and slow for 3-4 hours.

Scoop away the fat and any scum that rises to the surface once in a while.

After cooking, remove the bones and vegetables from the pot. Strain the broth. Let cool to room temperature and then put in the refrigerator.

The fat will solidify once the broth has chilled. Discard the fat (or reuse it) and pour the broth into a jar and freeze it.

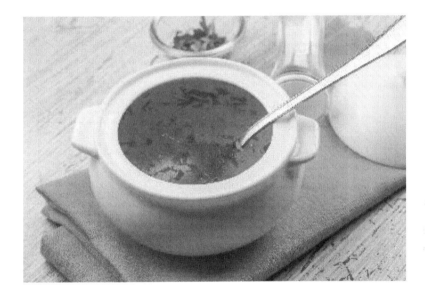

Pastes

Curry Paste

This should not be prepared in advance, but there are several curry recipes that are using curry paste and I decided to take the curry paste recipe out and have it separately. So, when you see that the recipe is using curry paste, please go to this part of the book and prepare it from scratch. Don't use processed curry pastes or curry powder; make it every time from scratch. Keep the spices in original form (seeds, pods), ground them just before making the curry paste. You can dry heat in the skillet cloves, cardamom, cumin and coriander and then crush them coarsely with mortar and pestle.

Ingredients

- 2 onions, minced
- 2 cloves garlic, minced
- 2 teaspoons fresh ginger root, finely chopped
- 6 whole cloves

- 2 cardamom pods
- 2 (2 inch) pieces cinnamon sticks, crushed
- 1 tsp. ground cumin
- 1 tsp. ground coriander
- 1 tsp. salt
- 1 tsp. ground cayenne pepper
- 1 tsp. ground turmeric

Instructions - Allergies: SF, GF, DF, EF, V, NF

Heat oil in a frying pan over medium heat and fry onions until transparent. Stir in garlic, cumin, ginger, cloves, cinnamon, coriander, salt, cayenne, and turmeric. Cook for 1 minute over medium heat, stirring constantly. At this point other curry ingredients should be added.

Tomato paste

Some recipes (chili) require tomato paste. I usually prepare 20 or so liters at once (when tomato is in season, which is usually September) and freeze it.

Ingredients

- 5 lbs. chopped plump tomatoes
- 1/4 cup extra-virgin <u>olive</u> oil or <u>avocado</u> oil plus 2 tbsp.
- salt, to taste

Instructions - Allergies: SF, GF, DF, EF, V, NF

Heat 1/4 cup of the oil in a skillet over medium heat. Add tomatoes. Season with salt. Bring to a boil. Cook, stirring, until very soft, about 8 minutes.

Pass the tomatoes through the finest plate of a food mill. Push as much of the pulp through the sieve as possible and leave the seeds behind.

Bring it to boil, lower it and then boil uncovered, so the liquid will thicken (approx. 30-40 minutes). That will give you homemade tomato juice. You get tomato paste if you boil for 60 minutes, it gets thick like store bought ketchup.

Store sealed in an airtight container in the refrigerator for up to one month, or freeze, for up to 6 months.

Precooked beans

Again, some recipes require that you cook some beans (butter beans, red kidney, garbanzo) in advance. Cooking beans takes around 3 hours and it can be done in advance or every few weeks and the rest get frozen. Soak beans for 24 hours before cooking them. After the first boil, throw the water, add new water and continue cooking. Some beans or lentils can be sprouted for few days before cooking and that helps people with stomach problems.

Breakfast - Oatmeal

Superfoods Oatmeal Breakfast
Allergies: SF, GF, DF, EF, V, NF

- 1/2 cup dry oatmeal
- 2 tsp. of ground <u>flax</u> seeds
- 2 tsp. of sunflower seeds
- A dash of cinnamon
- 1 tsp. of cocoa

Cook oatmeal with hot water and after that mix all ingredients. Sweeten if you have to with few drops of lucuma powder. Optional: You can replace sunflower seeds with pumpkin seed or chia seed. You can add a handful of blueberries or any berries instead of cocoa.

Oatmeal Yogurt Breakfast

Allergies: SF, GF, EF, NF

- 1/2 cup dry oatmeal

- Handful of blueberries (optional)

- 1 cups of low-fat yogurt

Mix all ingredients and wait 20 minutes or leave overnight in the fridge if using steel cut oats.

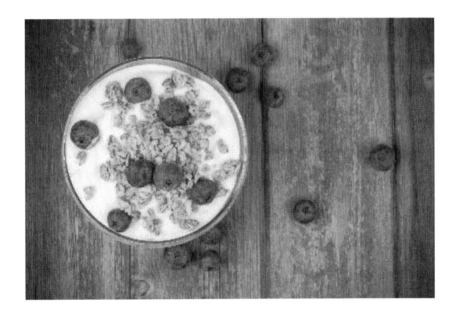

Cocoa Oatmeal

Ingredients - Allergies: SF, GF, DF, NF

- 1/2 cup dry oats
- 1 cup water
- A pinch tsp. salt
- 1/2 tsp. ground vanilla bean
- 1 tbsp. cocoa powder
- 1 tbsp. lucuma powder
- 3 tbsp. ground flax seeds meal
- a dash of cinnamon
- 2 egg whites

Instructions

In a saucepan over high heat, place the oats and salt. Cover with water. Bring to a boil and cook for 3-5 minutes, stirring occasionally. Keep adding 1/2 cup water if necessary as the mixture thickens.

In a separate bowl, whisk 4 tbsp. water into the 1 tbsp. cocoa powder to form a smooth sauce. Add the vanilla to the pan and stir.

Turn the heat down to low. Add the egg whites and whisk immediately. Add the flax meal, and cinnamon. Stir to combine. Remove from heat, add lucuma powder and serve immediately.

Topping suggestions: sliced strawberries, blueberries or few almonds.

Flax and Blueberry Vanilla Overnight Oats

Ingredients - Allergies: SF, GF, EF, V, NF

- 1/2 cup dry oats
- 1/3 cup water
- 1/2 cup low-fat yogurt
- 1/2 tsp. ground vanilla bean
- 2 tbsp. flax seeds meal
- A pinch of salt
- Blueberries, almonds, blackberries, lucuma powder for topping

Instructions

Add the ingredients (except for toppings) to the bowl in the evening. Refrigerate overnight.

In the morning, stir up the mixture. It should be thick. Add the toppings of your choice.

Apple Oatmeal

Ingredients - Allergies: SF, GF, DF, EF, V, NF

- 1/2 grated apple
- 1/2 cup dry oats
- 1 cups water
- Dash of cinnamon
- 1 tsp. lucuma powder

Instructions

Cook the oats with the water for 3-5 minutes.

Add grated apple and cinnamon. Stir in the lucuma powder.

Coconut Pomegranate Oatmeal

Ingredients - Allergies: SF, GF, DF, EF, V, NF

- 1/2 cup dry oats
- 1/3 cup coconut milk
- 1 cups water
- 2 tbs. shredded unsweetened coconut
- 1 tbs. flax seeds meal
- 1 tbs. lucuma powder
- 4 tbs. pomegranate seeds

Instructions

Cook oats with the coconut milk, water, and salt.

Stir in the coconut, lucuma powder and flaxseed meal. Sprinkle with extra coconut and pomegranate seeds.

Savory Breakfasts

Omelet with Leeks

Allergies: SF, GF, DF, NF

Cook 1 cup chopped leeks in little coconut oil until they get soft and then mix the 2 beaten eggs in.

Egg pizza crust

Ingredients - Allergies: SF, GF, DF, NF

- 2 eggs
- 1/4 cup of coconut flour
- 1/2 cup of coconut milk
- 1 small crushed garlic clove

Mix and make an omelet.

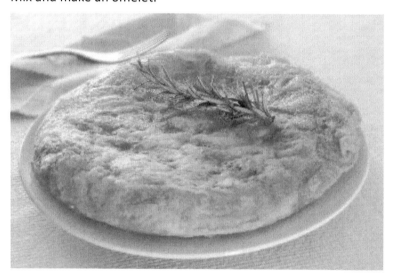

Omelet with Superfoods veggies

Ingredients - Allergies: SF, GF, DF, NF

- 2 large eggs
- Salt
- Ground black pepper
- 1 tsp. olive oil or cumin oil
- 1 cups spinach, cherry tomatoes and 1 spoon of yogurt cheese
- Crushed red pepper flakes and a pinch of dill (optional)

Instructions

Whisk 2 large eggs in a bowl. Season with salt and ground black pepper and set aside. Heat 1 tsp. olive oil in a medium skillet over medium heat. Add baby spinach, tomatoes, cheese and cook, tossing, until wilted (Approx. 1 minute). Add eggs; cook, stirring occasionally, until just set, about 1 minute. Stir in cheese. Sprinkle with crushed red pepper flakes and dill.

Egg Muffins

Ingredients - Allergies: SF, GF, DF, NF

Serving: 4 muffins

- 4 eggs
- 1/2 cup diced green bell pepper
- 1/2 cup diced onion
- 1/2 cup spinach
- 1/4 tsp. salt
- 1/8 tsp. ground black pepper
- 2 tbsp. water

Instructions

Heat the oven to 350 degrees F. Oil 4 muffin cups. Beat eggs together. Mix in bell pepper, spinach, onion, salt, black pepper, and water. Pour the mixture into muffin cups. Bake in the oven until muffins are done in the middle.

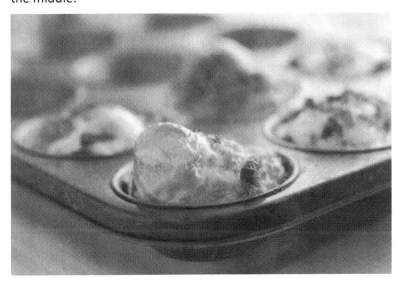

Smoked Salmon Scrambled Eggs

Ingredients - Allergies: SF, GF, DF, NF

- 1 tsp coconut oil
- 2 eggs
- 1 Tbs water
- 2 oz smoked salmon, sliced
- 1/4 avocado
- ground black pepper, to taste
- 2 chives, minced (or use 1 green onion, thinly sliced)

Instructions

Heat a skillet over medium heat. Add coconut oil to pan when hot. Meanwhile, scramble eggs. Add eggs to the hot skillet, along with smoked salmon. Stirring continuously, cook eggs until soft and fluffy. Remove from heat. Top with avocado, black pepper, and chives to serve.

Steak and Eggs

Ingredients - Allergies: SF, GF, DF, NF

- 1/4 lb boneless beef steak or pork tenderloin
- 1/4 tsp ground black pepper
- 1/4 tsp sea salt (optional)
- 1 tsp coconut oil
- 1/4 onion, diced
- 1/2 red bell pepper, diced
- 1 handful spinach or arugula
- 1 egg

Instructions

Season sliced steak or pork tenderloin with sea salt and black pepper. Heat a sauté pan over high heat. Add 1 tsp coconut oil, onions, and meat when pan is hot, and sauté until steak is slightly cooked. Add spinach and red bell pepper, and cook until steak is done to your liking. Meanwhile, heat a small fry pan over medium heat. Add remaining coconut oil, and fry two eggs. Top steak with a fried egg to serve.

Egg Bake

Ingredients - Allergies: SF, GF, DF, NF

- 1/2 cup chopped red peppers or spinach
- 1/4 cup zucchini
- 1/2 tbsp. coconut oil
- 1/4 cup sliced green onions
- 2 eggs
- 1/4 cup coconut milk
- 1/8 cup almond flour
- 1 tbsp. minced fresh parsley
- 1/4 tsp. dried basil
- 1/8 tsp. salt
- 1/8 tsp. ground black pepper

Instructions

Preheat oven to 350 degrees F. Put coconut oil in a skillet. Heat it to medium heat. Add mushrooms, onions, zucchini and red pepper (or spinach) until vegetables are tender, about 5 minutes. Drain veggies and spread them over the baking dish.

Beat eggs in a bowl with milk, flour, parsley, basil, salt, and pepper. Pour egg mixture into baking dish.

Bake in preheated oven until the center is set (approx. 35 to 40 minutes).

Frittata

Ingredients - Allergies: SF, GF, DF, NF

- 1 tbsp. <u>olive</u> oil or <u>avocado</u> oil
- 1/2 Zucchini, sliced
- 1/4 cup torn fresh spinach
- 1 tbsp. sliced green onions
- 1/4 tsp. crushed garlic, salt and pepper to taste
- 1/8 cup coconut milk
- 2 eggs

Instructions

Heat olive oil in a skillet over medium heat. Add zucchini and cook until tender. Mix in spinach, green onions, and garlic. Season with salt and pepper. Continue cooking until spinach is wilted.

 In a separate bowl, beat together eggs and coconut milk. Pour into the skillet over the vegetables. Reduce heat to low, cover, and cook until eggs are firm (5 to 7 minutes).

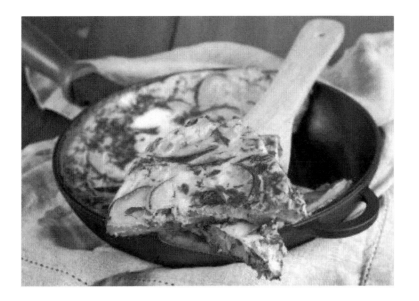

Superfoods Naan / Pancakes / Crepes

Ingredients - Allergies: SF, GF, DF, EF, V

- 1/2 cup <u>almond</u> flour
- 1/2 cup Tapioca Flour
- 1 cup Coconut Milk
- Salt
- <u>coconut oil</u>

Instructions

Mix all the ingredients together.

Heat a pan over medium heat and pour batter to desired thickness. Once the batter looks firm, flip it over to cook the other side.

If you want this to be a dessert crepe or pancake, then omit the salt. You can add minced garlic or ginger in the batter if you want, or some spices.

Zucchini Pancakes

Ingredients - Allergies: SF, GF, DF

- 1 small zucchini
- 1 tbsp. chopped onion
- 2 beaten eggs
- 3 tbsp. almond flour
- 1/2 tsp. salt
- 1/2 tsp. ground black pepper
- coconut oil

Instructions

Heat the oven to 300 degrees F.

Grate the zucchini into a bowl and stir in the onion and eggs. Stir in 6 tbsp. of the flour, salt, and pepper.

Heat a large sauté pan over medium heat and add coconut oil in the pan. When the oil is hot, lower the heat to medium-low and add batter into the pan. Cook the pancakes about 2 minutes on each side, until browned. Place the pancakes in the oven.

Superfoods Smoothies

Put the liquid in first. Surrounded by tea or yogurt, the blender blades can move freely. Next, add chunks of fruits or vegetables. Leafy greens are going into the pitcher last. Preferred liquid is green tea, but you can use almond or coconut milk or herbal tea.

Start slow. If your blender has speeds, start it on low to break up big pieces of fruit. Continue blending until you get a puree. If your blender can pulse, pulse a few times before switching to a puree mode. Once you have your liquid and fruit pureed, start adding greens, very slowly. Wait until previous batch of greens has been completely blended.

Thicken? Added too much tea or coconut milk? Thicken your smoothie by adding ice cubes, flax meal, chia seeds or oatmeal. Once you get used to various tastes of smoothies, add any seaweed, spirulina, chlorella powder or ginger for additional kick. Experiment with any Superfoods in powder form at this point. Think of adding any nut butter or sesame paste too or some Superfoods oils.

Rotate! Rotate your greens; don't always drink the same smoothie! At the beginning try 2 different greens every week and later introduce third and fourth one weekly. And keep rotating them. Don't use spinach and kale all the time. Try beets greens, they have a pinch of pink in them and that add great color to your smoothie. Here is the list of leafy green for you to try: spinach, kale, dandelion, chards, beet leaves, arugula, lettuce, collard greens, bok choy, cabbage, cilantro, parsley.

Flavor! Flavor smoothies with ground vanilla bean, cinnamon, lucuma powder, nutmeg, cloves, almond butter, cayenne pepper, ginger or just about any seeds or chopped nuts combination.

Not only are green smoothies high in nutrients, vitamins and fiber, they can also make any vegetable you probably don't like (be it kale, spinach or broccoli) taste great. The secret behind blending the perfect smoothie is using sweet fruits or nuts or seeds to give your drink a unique taste.

There's a reason kale and spinach seem to be the main ingredients in almost every green smoothie. Not only do they give smoothies their verdant color, they are also packed with calcium, protein and iron.

Although blending alone increases the accessibility of carotenoids, since the presence of fats is known to increase carotenoid absorption from leafy greens, it is possible that coconut oil, nuts and seeds in a smoothie could increase absorption further.

If you can't find some ingredient, replace it with the closest one.

GREEN SMOOTHIES

Kale Kiwi Smoothie

- 1 cup Kale, chopped

- 1 Apple

- 2 Kiwis

- 1 tablespoon flax seeds

- 1 tablespoon lucuma powder

- 1 cup crushed ice

Zucchini Apples Smoothie

- 1/2 cup zucchini

- 1 Apple

- 3/4 avocado

- 1 stalk Celery

- 1 Lemon

- 1 tbsp. Spirulina

- 1 1/2 cups crushed ice

Dandelion Smoothie

- 1 cup Dandelion greens

- 1 cup Spinach

- ½ cup tahini

- 1 Red Radish

- 1 tbsp. chia seeds

- 1 cup lavender tea

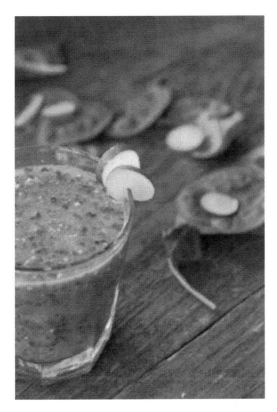

Broccoli Apple Smoothie

- 1 Apple

- 1 cup Broccoli

- 1 tbsp. Cilantro

- 1 Celery stalk

- 1 cup crushed ice

- 1 tbsp. crushed Seaweed

Salad Smoothie

- 1 cup spinach

- ½ cucumber

- 1/2 small onion

- 2 tablespoons Parsley

- 2 tablespoons lemon juice

- 1 cup crushed ice

- 1 tbsp. <u>olive</u> oil or <u>cumin</u> oil

- ¼ cup Wheatgrass

Avocado Kale Smoothie

- 1 cup Kale

- ½ Avocado

- 1 cup Cucumber

- 1 Celery Stalk

- 1 tbsp. chia seeds

- 1 cup chamomile tea

- 1 tbsp. Spirulina

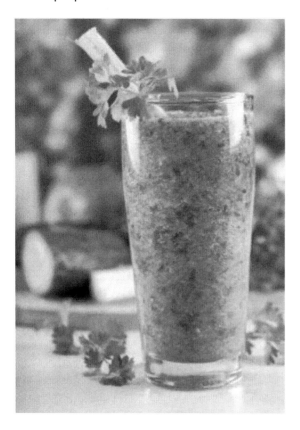

Watercress Smoothie

- 1 cup Watercress

- ½ cup <u>almond</u> butter

- 2 small cucumbers

- 1 cup coconut milk

- 1 tbsp. Chlorella

- 1 tbsp. Black cumin seeds – sprinkle on top and garnish with parsley

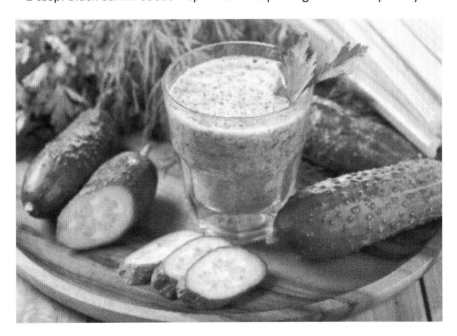

Beet Greens Smoothie

- 1 cup Beet Greens

- 2 tbsp. Pumpkin seeds butter

- 1 cup Strawberry

- 1 tbsp. Sesame seeds

- 1 tbsp. hemp seeds

- 1 cup chamomile tea

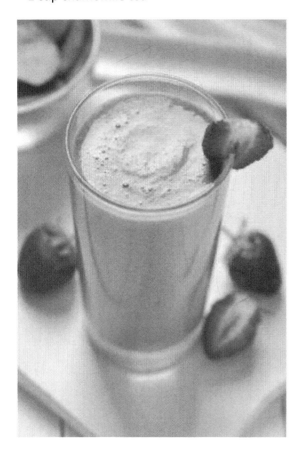

Broccoli Leeks Cucumber smoothie

- 1 cup Broccoli

- 2 tbsp. Cashew butter

- 2 Leeks

- 2 Cucumbers

- 1 Lime

- ½ cup Lettuce

- ½ cup Leaf Lettuce

- 1 tbsp. Matcha

- 1 cup crushed ice

Cacao Spinach Smoothie

- 2 cups spinach

- 1 cup blueberries, frozen

- 1 tablespoons dark cocoa powder

- ½ cup unsweetened almond milk

- 1/2 cup crushed ice

- 1 tsp lucuma powder

- 1 tbsp. Matcha powder

Flax Almond Butter Smoothie

- ½ cup plain yogurt

- 2 tablespoons almond butter

- 2 cups spinach

- 3 strawberries

- 1/2 cup crushed ice

- 1 teaspoon flax seeds

Apple Kale Smoothie

- 1 cup kale

- ½ cup coconut milk

- 1 tbsp. Maca

- ¼ teaspoon cinnamon

- 1 Apple

- Pinch of nutmeg

- 1 clove

- 3 ice cubes

Salad Dressings

Italian Dressing

Allergies: SF, GF, DF, EF, V, NF

- 2 tsp. olive oil or avocado oil
- lemon
- minced garlic
- salt

Yogurt Dressing

Allergies: SF, GF, DF, EF, V, NF

- 1 cup of plain low-fat Greek yogurt or low-fat buttermilk
- 1 tsp. olive oil or avocado oil
- minced garlic
- salt
- lemon

Occasionally I would add a tsp. of mustard or some herbs like basil, oregano, marjoram, chives, thyme, parsley, dill or mint. If you like spicy hot food, add some cayenne in the dressing. It will speed up your metabolism and have interesting hot spicy effect in cold yogurt or buttermilk.

Salads

Large Fiber Loaded Salad with Italian Dressing

Allergies: SF, GF, EF, NF

- 2 cups of spinach

- 1 cup of shredded cabbage, sauerkraut or lettuce. Cabbage has more substance.

- Italian or Yogurt dressing

- Cayenne pepper (optional)

- Few sprigs of cilantro (optional)

- 2 spring (green) onions (optional)

Large Fiber Loaded Salad with Yogurt Dressing

Serves 1 - Allergies: SF, GF, EF, NF

- 2 cups of spinach
- 1 cup of shredded cabbage or lettuce. Cabbage has more substance.
- Italian or Yogurt dressing
- Cayenne pepper (optional)
- Few sprigs of cilantro (optional)
- 2 spring (green) onions (optional)

Large Fiber Loaded Salad as a meal on its own

Allergies: SF, GF, EF, NF

This is what I eat every second evening and I can't get enough of it!!! This is the real secret to lose weight while having full stomach with grade A ingredients!!

- 2 cup of spinach

- 2 cup of shredded cabbage

- Yogurt dressing

- Cayenne pepper (optional)

- Few sprigs of cilantro (optional)

- 3 spring (green) onions

- 10 o.z. low-fat farmers' cheese

Pour yogurt dressing into the salad bowl. Add farmers' cheese and mix thoroughly. Cut spring onions in small pieces and add to the cheese mixture and mix. Add spinach and cabbage and mix thoroughly. Add spices (optional).

Greek Salad
Allergies: SF, GF, EF, NF

- 1 head romaine lettuce
- 1/2 lb. plump tomatoes
- 3 oz. Greek or black olives, sliced
- 2 oz. sliced radishes
- 4 oz. low-fat feta or goat cheese
- 2 oz. anchovies (optional)

Dressing:
- 2 oz. olive oil or avocado oil
- 2 oz. fresh lemon juice
- 1/2 tsp. dried oregano
- 1/4 tsp. black pepper
- 1/4 tsp. salt
- 2 cloves garlic, minced

Wash and cut lettuce into pieces. Slice tomatoes in quarters. Combine olives, lettuce, tomatoes, and radishes in large bowl. Mix dressing ingredients together and toss with vegetables. Pour out into a shallow serving bowl. Crumble feta/goat cheese over all, and arrange anchovy fillets on top (if desired).

Strawberry Spinach Salad

Ingredients - Allergies: SF, GF, DF, EF, V

- 1 tbsp. black sesame seeds
- 1 tbsp. poppy seeds
- 1/4 cup olive oil or cumin oil
- 1/8 cup lemon juice
- 1/8 tsp. paprika
- 1/2 bag fresh spinach - chopped, washed and dried
- 1 cup strawberries, sliced
- 1/4 cup toasted slivered almonds

Instructions

Whisk together the sesame seeds, olive oil, poppy seeds, paprika, lemon juice and onion. Refrigerate.
In a large bowl, combine the spinach, strawberries and almonds. Pour dressing over salad. Toss and refrigerate 15 minutes before serving.

Cucumber, Cilantro, Quinoa Tabbouleh

Serves 2

Ingredients - Allergies: SF, GF, DF, EF, NF, V

- 1/2 cup cooked quinoa mixed with 1 tbsp. sesame seeds
- 1/2 cup chopped tomato and green pepper
- 1 cup chopped cucumber
- 1/2 cup chopped cilantro

Dressing:
- 1 tbsp. olive oil or avocado oil
- 1 tbsp. fresh lemon juice
- pinch of black pepper
- pinch of sea salt

Instructions: Mix all ingredients.

Almond, Quinoa, Red Peppers & Arugula Salad

Serves 2

Ingredients - Allergies: SF, GF, DF, EF, NF, V

- 1/2 cup cooked <u>quinoa</u> mixed with 1 tbsp. pumpkin seeds
- 1/2 cup chopped almonds
- 1 cup chopped arugula
- 1/2 cup sliced red peppers

Dressing:
- 1 tbsp. <u>olive</u> oil or <u>cumin</u> oil
- 1 tbsp. fresh lemon juice
- pinch of black pepper
- pinch of sea salt

Instructions: Mix all ingredients.

Asparagus, Quinoa & Red Peppers Salad

Serves 2

Ingredients - Allergies: SF, GF, DF, EF, NF, V

- 1/2 cup cooked quinoa mixed with 1 tbsp. sunflower seeds
- 1 cup sliced red peppers
- 1 cup grilled asparagus
- Garnish with lime and parsley

Dressing:
- 1 tbsp. olive oil or avocado oil
- 1 tbsp. fresh lemon juice
- pinch of black pepper
- pinch of sea salt

Instructions: Mix all ingredients.

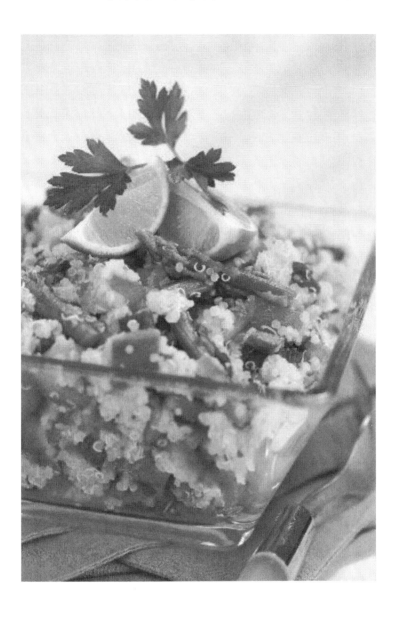

Chickpeas, Quinoa, Cucumber & Tomato Salad

Serves 2

Ingredients - Allergies: SF, GF, DF, EF, NF, V

- 1/2 cup cooked quinoa mixed with 1 tbsp. sesame seeds
- 1/2 cup cooked chickpeas
- 1 cup chopped cucumber and green onions
- 1/2 cup chopped tomato

Dressing:
- 1 tbsp. olive oil or avocado oil
- 1 tbsp. fresh lemon juice
- pinch of black pepper
- pinch of sea salt

Instructions: Mix all ingredients.

Quinoa Salad

Ingredients - Allergies: SF, GF, EF

For the salad

- 1/2 cup cooked quinoa
- 1/2 cup frozen green peas
- 1/4 cup low-fat feta cheese
- 4 oz. pork, cubed
- 1/8 cup freshly chopped basil and cilantro
- 1/8 cup almonds, pulsed in a food processor until crushed

For the dressing

- 1/8 cup lemon juice (1 juicy lemon)
- 1/8 cup olive oil or cumin oil
- 1/8 tsp. salt (more to taste)

Instructions

Bring a pot of water to boil and then lower the heat. Add the peas and cook covered until bright green. In the meantime, brown pork in a skillet. Toss the quinoa with the pork, peas, feta, herbs, and almonds.

Puree all the dressing ingredients in the food processor. Toss the dressing with the salad ingredients. Season generously with salt and pepper. Serve tossed with fresh baby spinach.

Cauliflower & Eggs Salad

Ingredients - Allergies: SF, GF, NF

- 1 cup chopped Cauliflower
- 2 hardboiled eggs - chopped,
- 2 oz. shredded cheddar cheese, low-fat
- 1/2 red onion, celery,
- 1 dill pickles,
- 1 tbsp. yellow mustard.

Mix all ingredients.

Greek Cucumber Salad

Ingredients - Allergies: SF, GF, EF, NF

- 2 cucumbers, sliced
- 1 teaspoon salt
- 2 tbsp. lemon juice
- 1/4 tsp. paprika
- 1/4 tsp. white pepper
- 1/2 clove garlic, minced
- 2 fresh green onions, diced
- 1 cup thick Greek Yogurt

- 1/4 tsp. paprika

Instructions

Slice cucumbers thinly, sprinkle with salt and mix. Set aside for one hour. Mix lemon juice, water, garlic, paprika and white pepper, and set aside. Squeeze liquid from cucumber slices a few at a time, and place slices in the bowl. Discard liquid. Add lemon juice mixture, green onions, and yogurt. Mix and sprinkle additional paprika or dill over top. Chill for 1-2 hours.

Mediterranean Salad

Ingredients - Allergies: SF, GF, DF, EF, V, NF

- 1 small head romaine lettuce, torn
- 1 tomato, diced
- 1 small cucumber, sliced
- 1/2 green bell pepper, sliced
- 1/2 small onion, cut into rings
- 3 radishes, thinly sliced
- 1/4 cup flat leaf parsley, chopped
- 1/4 cup <u>olive</u> oil or <u>avocado</u> oil
- 2 tbsp. lemon juice
- 1 garlic clove, minced
- Salt & pepper
- 1 tsp. fresh mint, minced

Instructions

Combine lettuce, tomatoes, cucumber, pepper, onion, radishes & parsley in a salad bowl. Whisk together olive oil, lemon juice, garlic, salt, pepper & mint. Pour over salad & toss to coat.

Pomegranate Avocado salad

Ingredients - Allergies: SF, GF, DF, EF, V

- 2 cups mixed greens, spinach, arugula, red leaf lettuce
- 1 ripe avocado, cut into 1/2-inch pieces
- 1 cup pomegranate seeds
- 1/2 cup pecan
- 1/2 cup blackberries
- 1/2 cup cherry tomatoes
- Olive oil, salt, lemon juice

Instructions

Combine greens, pecan, cut avocado, tomatoes, pomegranates and blackberries in a salad bowl. Whisk together salt, olive oil and lemon juice and pour over salad.

Roasted Beet Salad

Instructions - Allergies: SF, GF, DF, EF, V, NF

Toss 3 beets cut in half in a baking dish with olive oil, salt and pepper. Cover and roast at 425 degrees F until tender; let cool, then rub off the skins. Toss with any juices from the baking dish, capers, chopped pickles, a dash each of hot sauce, and chopped parsley or dill.

Apple Coleslaw

Ingredients - Allergies: SF, GF, DF, EF, V, NF

- 2 cups chopped cabbage (various color)
- 1 tart apple chopped
- 1 celery, chopped
- 1 red pepper chopped
- 4 tsp. <u>olive</u> oil or <u>avocado</u> oil
- juice of 1 lemon
- 1 Tbs. lucuma powder (optional)
- dash sea salt

Instructions

Toss the cabbage, apple, celery, and pepper together in a large bowl. In a smaller bowl, whisk remaining ingredients. Drizzle over coleslaw and toss to coat.

Carrot, Quinoa, Tomato & Spinach Salad in a Jar
Serves 2

Ingredients - Allergies: SF, GF, EF, NF

- 1/2 cup sunflower seeds and 1/2 cup carrots
- 1/2 cup of shredded cabbage and 1/2 cup of tomatoes
- 1 cup cooked quinoa mixed with 1 tbsp. chia seeds
- 1 cup spinach

Dressing:

- 1 tbsp. olive oil
- 1 tbsp. fresh lemon juice and pinch of sea salt

Instructions: Put ingredients in this order: dressing, sunflower seeds, carrots, cabbage, tomatoes and spinach.

Chickpeas, Onion, Tomato & Parsley Salad in a Jar
Serves 2

Ingredients - Allergies: SF, GF, EF, NF

- 1 cup cooked chickpeas
- 1/2 cup chopped tomatoes
- 1/2 of a small onion, chopped
- 1 tbsp. chia seeds
- 1 Tbsp. chopped parsley

Dressing:

- 1 tbsp. olive oil and 1 tbsp. of Chlorella.
- 1 tbsp. fresh lemon juice and pinch of sea salt

Instructions: Put ingredients in this order: dressing, tomatoes, chickpeas, onions and parsley.

Arugula, Carrot, Corn & Spinach Salad in a Jar
Serves 2

Ingredients - Allergies: SF, GF, EF, NF

- 1 cup corn
- 1 cup tomatoes
- 1/2 cup of julienned carrot
- 1/2 cup spinach

Dressing:

- 1 tbsp. olive oil and 2 Tbsp. Greek Yogurt
- 1 tbsp. fresh lemon juice and pinch of sea salt

Instructions: Put ingredients in this order: dressing, tomatoes, corn, carrots, and arugula.

Shrimp, Cucumber & Arugula Salad in a Jar

Serves 2

Ingredients - Allergies: SF, GF, EF, NF

- 1 cup cooked shrimp
- 1/2 cup of cucumber
- 1 cup of arugula

Dressing:

- 1 tbsp. <u>olive</u> oil
- 1 tbsp. fresh lemon juice and pinch of sea salt

Instructions: Put ingredients in this order: dressing, cucumber, shrimp and arugula.

Tomato, Cucumber, Pumpkin & Dandelion Jar Salad

Serves 2

Ingredients - Allergies: SF, GF, EF, NF

- 1/2 cup cooked, cubed pumpkin
- 1/2 cup tomatoes
- 1/2 cup of sliced cucumber
- 1/2 cup Dandelion leaves

Dressing:

- 1 tbsp. olive oil and 1 tbsp. of Chlorella
- 1 tbsp. fresh lemon juice and pinch of sea salt

Instructions: Put ingredients in this order: dressing, tomatoes, cucumbers, pumpkin and dandelion leaves.

Carrot, Peppers, Cucumber & Cabbage Salad in a Jar
Serves 2

Ingredients - Allergies: SF, GF, EF, NF

- 1/2 cup chopped cucumber and 1/2 cup chopped carrots
- 1/2 cup of shredded red cabbage and 1/2 cup of red peppers
- 1 cup lettuce

Dressing:
- 1 tbsp. olive oil
- 1 tbsp. fresh lemon juice and pinch of sea salt

Instructions: Put ingredients in this order: dressing, cucumbers, peppers, cabbage, carrots and lettuce.

Tomato, Cucumber, Carrot & Parsley Salad in a Jar
Serves 2

Ingredients - Allergies: SF, GF, EF, NF

- 1/2 cup red tomatoes
- 1/2 cup yellow tomatoes
- 1/2 cup of sliced carrot
- 1 Tbsp. of chopped parsley

Dressing:

- 1 tbsp. olive oil and 2 Tbsp. Greek Yogurt
- 1 tbsp. fresh lemon juice and pinch of sea salt

Instructions: Put ingredients in this order: dressing, cucumbers, yellow tomato, carrots, red tomato and parsley.

Watercress, Cabbage & Carrot Salad in a Jar

Serves 2

Ingredients - Allergies: SF, GF, EF, NF

- 1/2 cup shredded green cabbage
- 1/2 cup of shredded red cabbage
- 1/2 cup julienned carrots
- 1 cup watercress

Dressing:

- 1 tbsp. olive oil
- 1 tbsp. fresh lemon juice and pinch of sea salt

Instructions: Put ingredients in this order: dressing, green cabbage, red cabbage, carrots and watercress.

Chickpeas, Tomato & Peppers Salad in a Jar
Serves 2

Ingredients - Allergies: SF, GF, EF, NF

- 3/4 cup chickpeas
- 1/2 cup tomatoes &1/2 cup of dandelion leaves
- 1/2 cup of sliced cucumber
- 1/2 cup of yellow pepper

Dressing:
- 1 tbsp. olive oil and 2 Tbsp. Greek Yogurt
- 1 tbsp. fresh lemon juice and pinch of sea salt

Instructions: Put ingredients in this order: dressing, cucumber, tomato, chickpeas, peppers and dandelion leaves.

Soups

Cream of Broccoli Soup

Ingredients - Allergies: SF, GF, EF, NF

- 1 pound broccoli, fresh
- 1 cup water
- 1/4 tsp. salt, pepper to taste
- 1/4 cup tapioca flour, mixed with 1 cup cold water
- 1/4 cup coconut cream
- 1/4 cup low-fat farmers' cheese

Steam or boil broccoli until it gets tender.
Put 1 cup of water and coconut cream in top of double boiler.
Add salt, cheese and pepper. Heat until cheese gets melted.
Add broccoli. Mix water and tapioca flour in a small bowl.
Stir tapioca mixture into cheese mixture in double boiler and heat until soup thickens.

Lentil Soup

Ingredients - Allergies: SF, GF, DF, EF, NF
- 1 tbsp. <u>olive</u> oil or <u>avocado</u> oil
- 1/2 cup finely chopped onion
- 1/4 cup chopped carrot
- 1/4 cup chopped celery
- 1 teaspoons salt
- 1/2 pound lentils
- 1/2 cup chopped tomatoes
- 1 quart chicken or vegetable broth
- 1/4 tsp. ground coriander & toasted cumin

Instructions

Place the olive oil into a large Dutch oven. Set over medium heat. Once hot, add the celery, onion, carrot and salt and do until the onions are translucent. Add the lentils, tomatoes, cumin, broth and coriander and stir to combine. Increase the heat and bring just to a boil. Reduce the heat, cover and simmer at a low until the lentils are tender (approx. 35 to 40 minutes). Puree with a bender to your preferred consistency (optional). Serve immediately.

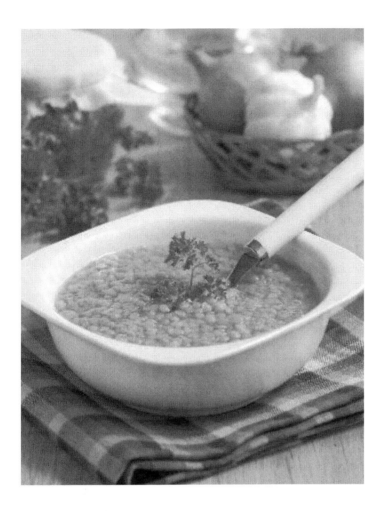

Cold Cucumber Avocado Soup

Ingredients - Allergies: SF, GF, EF, NF
- 1 cucumber peeled, seeded and cut into 2-inch chunks
- 1 avocado, peeled
- 1 chopped scallions
- 1 cup chicken broth
- 1/3 cup Greek low-fat yogurt
- 1 tbsp. lemon juice
- 1/4 tsp. ground pepper, or to taste

Garnish:
- Chopped chives, dill, mint, scallions or cucumber

Instructions

Combine the cucumber, avocado and scallions in a blender. Pulse until chopped.

Add yogurt, broth and lemon juice and continue until smooth.

Season with pepper and salt to taste and chill for 4 hours.

Taste for seasoning and garnish.

Bouillabaisse

Ingredients - Allergies: SF, GF, DF, EF, NF

- 1 pound of 3 different kinds of fish fillets
- 1/4 cup Coconut oil
- 1 pounds of Oysters, clams, or mussels
- 1/3 cup cooked shrimp, crab, or lobster meat, or rock lobster tails
- 1/3 cup thinly sliced onions
- 1 Shallot or the white parts of 1 leek, thinly sliced
- 1 cloves garlic, crushed
- 1 small tomato, chopped
- 1/2 sweet red pepper, chopped
- 2 stalks celery, thinly sliced
- 1-inch slice of fennel or 1/2 tsp. of fennel seed
- 1 sprigs fresh thyme or 1/4 tsp. dried thyme
- 1 bay leaf
- 1 whole cloves
- Zest of half an orange
- 1/4 tsp. saffron
- 1 teaspoons salt
- 1/4 tsp. ground black pepper
- 1/3 cup clam juice or fish broth
- 1 Tbps lemon juice
- 1/3 cup white wine

Instructions

In a large saucepan heat 1/8 cup of the coconut oil. When it is hot, add onions and shallots (or leeks). Sauté for a minute. Add crushed garlic, and sweet red pepper. Add celery, tomato, and fennel. Stir the vegetables until well coated. Add another 1/8 cup of coconut oil, bay leaf, thyme, cloves and the orange zest. Cook until the onion is golden. Cut fish fillets into 2-inch pieces. Add 1 cup of water and the pieces of fish to the vegetable mixture. Bring to a boil, then reduce heat and let it simmer, uncovered, for about 10 minutes. Add clams, oysters or mussels (optional) and crabmeat, shrimp or lobster tails, cut into pieces. Add salt, saffron and pepper. Add lemon juice, clam juice, and white wine. Bring to a simmer again and cook for 5 minutes longer.

Gaspacho

Ingredients - Allergies: SF, GF, DF, EF, V, NF
- 1/4 cup of flax seeds meal
- 1 pound tomatoes, diced
- 1 red pepper or 1 green pepper, diced
- 1 small cucumber, peeled and diced
- 1 cloves of garlic, peeled and crushed
- ¼ cup extra virgin olive oil or cumin oil
- 1 tbsp. lemon juice
- Salt, to taste

Instructions
Mix the peppers, tomatoes and cucumber with the crushed garlic and olive oil in the bowl of a blender. Add flax meal to the mixture. Blend until smooth. Add salt and lemon juice to taste and stir well. Refrigerate. Serve with black olives, hard-boiled egg, cilantro, mint or parsley.

Italian Beef Soup

Ingredients - Allergies: SF, GF, DF, EF, NF

- 1/3 pound minced beef
- 1 clove garlic, minced
- 1 cups beef broth
- 1 large tomato
- 1/2 cup sliced carrots
- 1/2 cup cooked beans
- 1 small zucchini, cubed
- 1 cups spinach - rinsed and torn
- 1/8 tsp. black pepper
- 1/8 tsp. salt

Brown beef with garlic in a stockpot. Stir in broth, carrots and tomatoes. Season with salt and pepper. Reduce heat, cover, and simmer for 15 minutes.
Stir in beans with liquid and zucchini. Cover, and simmer until zucchini is tender. Remove from heat, add spinach and cover. Serve after 5 minutes.

Creamy roasted mushroom

Ingredients - Allergies: SF, GF, DF, EF, V, NF

- 1/2 pound Portobello mushrooms, cut into 1inch pieces
- 1/4 pound shiitake mushrooms, stemmed
- 2 tbsp. olive oil or avocado oil
- 1 cups vegetable broth
- 1 tbsp. coconut oil
- 1/2 onion, chopped
- 1 garlic cloves, minced
- 1 tbsp. arrowroot flour
- 1/4 cup coconut cream
- 1/4 tsp. chopped thyme

Instructions

Heat oven to 400°F. Line one large baking sheets with foil. Spread mushrooms and drizzle some olive oil on them. Season with salt and pepper and toss. Cover with foil and bake them for half an hour. Uncover and continue baking 15 minutes more. Cool slightly. Mix one half of the mushrooms with one can of broth in a blender. Set aside.

Melt coconut oil in a large pot over high heat. Add onion and garlic and sauté until onion is translucent. Add flour and stir 2 minutes. Add cream, broth, and thyme. Stir in remaining cooked mushrooms and mushroom puree. Simmer over low heat until thickened (approx. 10 minutes). Season to taste with salt and pepper.

Black Bean Soup

Ingredients - Allergies: SF, GF, DF, EF, NF

- 1 Tbsp. cup Coconut Oil
- 1/4 cup Onion, Diced
- 1/4 cup Carrots, Diced
- 1/4 cup Green Bell Pepper, Diced
- 1 cup beef broth
- 1 pound cooked Black Beans
- 1 tbsp. lemon juice
- 1 teaspoons chopped Garlic
- 1 teaspoons Salt
- 1/4 tsp. Black Pepper, Ground
- 1 teaspoons Chili Powder
- 4 oz. pork
- 1 tbsp. tapioca flour
- 2 tbsp. Water

Instructions

Place coconut oil, onion, carrot, and bell pepper in a stock pot. Cook the veggies until tender. Bring broth to a boil. Add cooked beans, broth and the remaining ingredients (except tapioca flour and 2 tbsp. water) to the vegetables. Bring that mixture to a simmer and cook approximately 15 minutes. Puree 1 quart of the soup in a blender and put back into the pot. Combine the tapioca flour and 2 tbsp. water in a separate bowl. Add the tapioca flour mixture to the bean soup and bring to a boil for 1 minute.

Squash soup

Ingredients - Allergies: SF, GF, DF, EF, V, NF

• 1 small squash

• 1 carrot, chopped

• 1/2 onion (diced)

• 1/2 cup coconut milk

• 1/4 cup water

• 1 tbsp. olive oil or avocado oil

• Salt

• Pepper

• Cinnamon

• Turmeric

Instructions

Cut the squash and spoon out the seeds. Cut it into large pieces and place on a baking sheet. Sprinkle with salt, olive oil, and pepper and bake at 375 degrees F until soft (approx. 1 hour). Let cool.

In the meantime, sauté the onions in olive oil (put it in a soup pot). Add the carrots. Add 1/4 cup coconut milk and 1/4 cup water after few minutes and let simmer. Scoop the squash out of its skin. Add it to the soup pot. Stir to combine the ingredients and let simmer a few minutes. Add more milk or water if needed. Season to taste with the salt, pepper and spices. Blend until smooth and creamy.

Sprinkle it with toasted pumpkin seeds.

Kale White Bean Pork Soup

Ingredients - Allergies: SF, GF, DF, EF, NF

- 1 tbsp. each extra-virgin olive oil and <u>coconut oil</u>
- 1 tbsp. chili powder
- 1/2 tbsp. jalapeno hot sauce
- 1/2 pound bone-in pork chops
- Salt
- 2 stalks celery, chopped
- 1 small white onion, chopped
- 1 cloves garlic, chopped
- 1 cup chicken broth
- 1 cups diced tomatoes
- 1/2 cup cooked white beans
- 2 cups packed Kale

Instructions

Preheat the broiler. Whisk hot sauce, 1 tbsp. olive oil and a pinch of chili powder in a bowl. Season the pork chops with 1/2 tsp. salt. Rub chops with the spice mixture on both sides and place them on a rack set over a baking sheet. Set aside.

Heat 1 tbsp. coconut oil in a large pot over high heat. Add the celery, garlic, onion and the remaining chili powder. Cook until onions are translucent, stirring (approx. 8 minutes).

Add tomatoes and the chicken broth to the pot. Cook and stir occasionally until reduced by about one-third (approx. 7 minutes). Add the kale and the beans. Reduce the heat to medium, cover and cook until the kale is tender (approx. 7 minutes). Add up to 1/2 cup water if the mixture looks dry and season with salt.

In the meantime, broil the pork until browned (approx. 4 to 6 minutes). Flip and broil until cooked through. Serve with the kale and beans.

Avgolemono – Greek lemon chicken soup

Ingredients - Allergies: SF, GF, DF, EF, NF

• 2 cups chicken broth

• 1/4 cup uncooked quinoa

• salt and pepper

• 2 eggs

• 2 tbsp. lemon juice

• Handful fresh dill (chopped)

• shredded roasted chicken (optional)

Bring the broth to a boil in a saucepan. Add the quinoa and cook until tender. Season with the salt and pepper. Reduce heat to low and let simmer. In a separate bowl, whisk lemon juice and the eggs until smooth. Add about 1 cup of the hot broth into the egg/lemon mixture and whisk to combine.

Add the mixture back to the saucepan. Stir until the soup becomes opaque and thickens. Add dill, salt and pepper. Optionally add chicken and serve.

Egg-Drop Soup

Ingredients - Allergies: SF, GF, DF, NF

• 2 cups quarts chicken broth
• 1 tbsps. Tapioca flour, mixed in 1/4 cup cold water
• 2 eggs, slightly beaten with a fork
• 2 scallions, chopped, including green ends

Instructions

Bring broth to a boil. Slowly pour in the tapioca flour mixture while stirring the broth. The broth should thicken. Reduce heat and let it simmer. Mix in the eggs very slowly while stirring. As soon as the last drop of egg is in, turn off the heat. Serve with chopped scallions on top.

Creamy Tomato Basil Soup

Ingredients - Allergies: SF, GF, DF, EF, V, NF

- 2 tomatoes - peeled, seeded and diced
- 2 cups tomato juice*
- 5 leaves fresh basil
- 1/2 cup coconut cream
- salt to taste
- ground black pepper to taste

Instructions

Combine tomatoes and tomato juice in stock pot. Simmer 30 minutes. Puree mixture with basil leaves in a processor. Put back in a stock pot and add coconut cream. Add salt and pepper to taste.

Minestrone

Ingredients - Allergies: SF, GF, DF, EF, NF

- 1 tbsp. coconut oil
- 1 cloves garlic, chopped
- 1/2 onions, chopped
- 1/2 cups chopped celery
- 2 carrots, sliced
- 1 cup chicken broth
- 1/2 cups water
- 1 cup tomato sauce
- 1/2 oz. red wine (optional)
- 1/2 cup cooked kidney beans
- 1/2 cups green beans
- 1/2 cups baby spinach, rinsed
- 1 small zucchinis, quartered and sliced
- 1/2 tbsp. chopped oregano
- 1 tbsp. chopped basil
- salt and pepper to taste
- 1/2 tbsp. olive oil or cumin oil

Instructions

Heat coconut oil over medium heat in a stock pot, and sauté garlic for few minutes. Add onion and sauté for few more minutes. Add celery and carrots and sauté for 2 minutes.

Add chicken broth, tomato sauce and water and bring to boil, stirring frequently. Add red wine at this point. Reduce heat to low and add kidney beans, zucchini, green beans, spinach leaves, oregano, basil, salt and pepper. Simmer for 30 to 40 minutes.

Grilled Meats & Salad

Chicken and Large Fiber Loaded Salad with Italian Dressing

Allergies: SF, GF, EF, NF

• 2 6oz. pieces of Chicken (or turkey), skinless, boneless grilled or prepared in the skillet.

• Large mixed spinach and lettuce salad with Italian Dressing and half a tsp of mustard. Salad can be as large as you want, but use half a cup of the dressing.

Salmon with Large Fiber Loaded Salad with Italian Dressing

Allergies: SF, GF, DF, EF, NF

• 2 Salmon steaks grilled or prepared in the skillet.

• Large mixed spinach and lettuce salad with "Italian Dressing" and some thyme sprinkled on top of it. Salad can be as large as you want, but use the prescribed amount of the dressing.

Ground Beef Patty with Large Fiber Loaded Salad with Yogurt Dressing

Allergies: SF, GF, EF, NF

• 2 5oz. lean ground beef patty grilled or prepared in the skillet.

• Large mixed spinach and shredded cabbage salad with Yogurt Dressing. Salad can be as large as you want, but use half a cup of a dressing.

Lean Pork with Fiber Loaded Salad with Yogurt Dressing

Allergies: SF, GF, EF, NF

- 2 5oz. lean Pork Tenderloin pieces grilled or prepared in the skillet.

- Large mixed spinach and shredded cabbage salad with Yogurt Dressing and half a tsp of mustard. Salad can be as large as you want, but use half a cup of the dressing.

Caribbean Chicken salad

Ingredients - Allergies: SF, GF, DF, EF, NF

2 boneless skinless chicken breasts

Marinade

1/2 cup fish sauce

2 tomatoes (seeded and chopped)

1/2 cup chopped onion

2 tsps. jalapeno chilies (minced)

2 tsps. chopped cilantro fresh

Lucuma powder Lime Dressing:

1/4 cup mustard

1/4 cup lucuma powder

1 tbsp coconut oil

1 1/2 tbsps. lemon juice

1 1/2 tsps. lime juice

3/4 lb mixed greens

Instructions

Blend all the marinade ingredients in a small bowl with a hand blender. Cover and chill. Marinate the chicken for at least two hours in the fridge. Grill the chicken for few minutes per side or until done.

Serve the greens into 2 large salad bowls.
Slice the chicken into thin strips. Divide among bowls.
Pour the dressing aside and serve with the salads.

Herb Crusted Salmon

Allergies: SF, GF, DF, EF, NF

Rub some tarragon, chives and parsley over 2 salmon steaks and add some salt and pepper. Heat the pan with 1 tsp of coconut oil to medium high and place the salmon, skin-side up in the pan. Cook until golden brown on 1 side, about 4 minutes. Turn the fish over and cook until it feels firm to the touch. Salmon is done when it flakes easily with a fork. Serve with a wedge of lemon.

• Large mixed spinach and lettuce salad with "Italian Dressing" and some thyme sprinkled on top of it. Salad can be as large as you want, but use the prescribed amount of the dressing.

Tuna with Large Fiber Loaded Salad with Italian Dressing

Allergies: SF, GF, DF, EF, NF

- 2 6oz. can of Tuna, drained.

- Large mixed spinach and green onion salad with Italian Dressing and half a tsp of mustard. Salad can be as large as you want, but use only the prescribed amount of dressing. You may use fish sauce instead of salt.

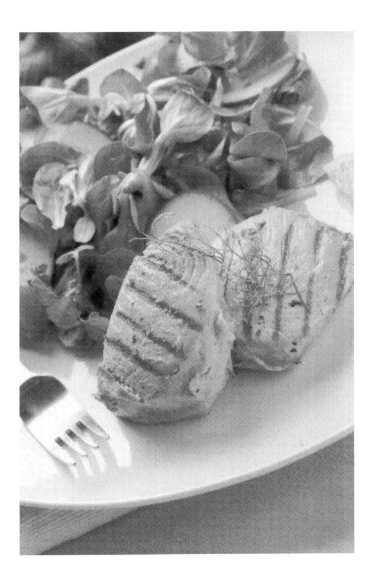

Stews, Chilies and Curries

Vegetarian Chili

Ingredients - Allergies: SF, GF, DF, EF, V, NF

1 tbsp. coconut oil
1/2 cup chopped onions
1/2 cup chopped carrots
1 cloves garlic, minced
1/2 cup chopped green bell pepper
1/2 cup chopped red bell pepper
1/4 cup chopped celery
1/2 tbsp. chili powder
1/2 cups chopped mushrooms
1 cup chopped tomatoes
1 cups cooked kidney beans
1/2 tbsp. ground cumin
1/2 teaspoons oregano
1/2 teaspoons crushed basil leaves

Instructions

Heat coconut oil in a large saucepan and add onions, carrots and garlic; sauté until tender. Stir in green pepper, red pepper, celery and chili powder.
Cook, stirring often, until vegetables are tender, about 6 minutes. To the vegetables add mushrooms; cook 4 minutes. Stir in tomatoes, kidney beans, corn, cumin, oregano and basil. Bring to a boil. Reduce heat to medium. Cover and simmer for 20 minutes, stirring occasionally.

Lentil Stew

Ingredients - Allergies: SF, GF, DF, EF, NF

- 1 cup dry lentils
- 2 cups chicken broth
- 1 tomato
- 1/4 cup chopped carrot
- 1/4 cup chopped onion + 1/4 cup chopped celery (optional)
- few sprigs of parsley and basil + 1 garlic clove (minced)
- 1/2 pound of cubed lean pork or beef + pepper to taste

You can eat a salad of your choice with this stew.

Braised Green Peas with Beef

Ingredients - Allergies: SF, GF, DF, EF, NF

- 2 cups fresh or frozen green peas

- 1 onion, finely chopped

- 2 cloves of garlic, thinly sliced and 1/2 inch of peeled/sliced fresh ginger (if you like)

- 1/2 tsp. red pepper flakes, or to taste

- 1 tomato, roughly chopped

- 2 chopped carrots

- 2 tbsp. coconut oil

- 1 cup chicken broth

- 10 oz. cubed beef

- Salt and freshly ground black pepper

Heat the coconut oil in a skillet over medium heat. Sauté the onion, garlic and ginger until they are soft. Add the red pepper, carrot, and tomatoes and sauté until the tomato begins to soften. Add in the green peas. Add cubed lean beef. Add in the broth and simmer over medium heat. Cover and cook until the peas are tender. Season to taste with salt and pepper.

White Chicken Chili

Ingredients - Allergies: SF, GF, DF, EF, NF

- 2 large boneless, skinless chicken breasts
- 1 green bell peppers
- 1/2 yellow onion
- 1/2 jalapeno
- 1/4 cup diced green chilies (optional)
- 1/4 cup of spring onions
- 1 tbsp. coconut oil
- 1/2 cup cooked white beans
- 2 cups chicken or vegetable broth
- 1/2 tsp. ground cumin
- 1/8 tsp. cayenne pepper
- salt to taste

Instructions

Bring a pot of water to boil. Add the chicken breasts and cook until cooked through. Drain water and allow chicken to cool. When cool, shred and set aside.

Dice the bell peppers, jalapeno and onion. Melt the coconut oil in a pot over high heat. Add the peppers and onions and sauté until soft, approx. 8-10 minutes.

Add the broth, beans, chicken and spices to the pot. Stir and bring to a low boil. Cover and simmer for 25-30 minutes.

Simmer for 10 more minutes and stir occasionally. Remove from heat. Let stand for 10 minutes to thicken. Top with cilantro.

Kale Pork

Ingredients - Allergies: SF, GF, DF, EF, NF

- 1 tbsp. <u>coconut oil</u>
- 1/2 pound pork tenderloin, trimmed and cut into 1-inch pieces
- 1/4 tsp. salt
- 1/2 medium onion, finely chopped
- 2 cloves garlic, minced
- 1 teaspoons paprika
- 1/8 tsp. crushed red pepper (optional)
- 1/2 cup white wine
- 2 plump tomatoes, chopped
- 2 cups chicken broth
- 1/2 bunch kale, chopped
- 1 cups cooked white beans

Instructions

Heat oil in a pot over medium heat. Add pork, season with salt and cook until no longer pink. Transfer to a plate and leave juices in the pot.

Add onion to the pot and cook until turns translucent. Add paprika, garlic and crushed red pepper and cook about 30 seconds. Add tomatoes and wine, increase heat and stir to scrape up any browned bits. Add broth. Bring to a boil.

Add kale and stir until it wilts. Lower the heat and simmer, until the kale is tender. Stir in beans, pork and pork juices. Simmer for 2 more minutes.

30-Minute Squash Cauliflower and Green Peppers Coconut Curry

Ingredients - Allergies: SF, GF, DF, EF, V, NF

- Curry Paste
- 1 cups peeled, chopped squash
- 1 cup thick coconut milk
- 1 tbsp. coconut oil
- 1 tbsp. lucuma powder
- 1 pound tomatoes
- 1/2 cup brown rice, uncooked
- 1/2 cup chopped Cauliflower
- 1/2 cup chopped Green Peppers
- Cilantro for topping

Instructions

Cook brown rice. Set aside.

Make Curry Paste. Pour the coconut milk into the skillet and mix the curry and lucuma powder into the coconut milk. Add the cauliflower, squash, and green peppers. Cover and simmer until squash is tender. Remove from heat and let stand for 10 minutes. The sauce will thicken.

Serve the curry with chopped cilantro.

Crockpot Red Curry Lamb

Ingredients - Allergies: SF, GF, DF, EF, NF

- 1/2 pounds cubed lamb meat
- Curry Paste *
- 1/2 cups tomato paste
- 1 tsp. salt
- 1/4 cup coconut milk or cream

Instructions

Make the Curry Paste. Add lamb and the curry paste in a crockpot. Pour half a cup of tomato paste over the lamb. Add 1/4 cups of water to the crockpot. Stir, cover and cook on high for 2 hours or low for 4-5 hours. Taste and season with salt.

Stir in the coconut milk and sprinkle with cilantro before serving.

Easy Lentil Dhal

Ingredients - Allergies: SF, GF, DF, EF, V, NF

- 1 cup lentils
- 1 cup of water
- Curry Paste *
- 1/4 cup coconut milk
- 1/4 cup water
- 1/4 teaspoons salt + 1/8 tsp. black pepper
- lime juice
- Cilantro and spring onions for garnish

Instructions

Bring the water to a boil in a large pot. Add lentils and cook uncovered for 10 minutes, stirring frequently. Remove from heat. Stir in remaining ingredients. Season with salt and herbs for garnish.

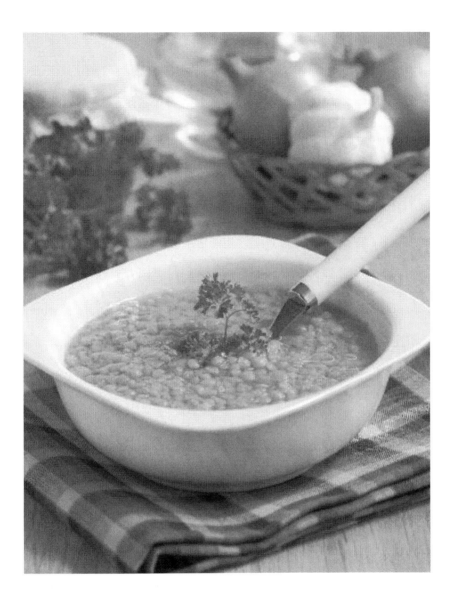

Gumbo

Ingredients - Allergies: SF, GF, DF, EF, NF

- 1/4 pound medium shrimp peeled
- 1/4 pound skinless, boneless chicken breasts, cut bite size
- 1 Tbsp. coconut oil
- 1 Tbsp. almond flour
- 1/2 cups chopped onions
- 1/4 cup chopped celery
- 1/4 cup chopped green pepper
- 1/4 tsp. ground cumin
- 1/4 tbsp. minced fresh garlic
- 1/4 tsp. fresh thyme chopped
- 1/8 tsp. red pepper
- 1 cup chicken broth
- 1/2 cups diced tomatoes
- 1/2 cups sliced okra
- 1/4 cup fresh parsley chopped
- 1 bay leaf
- 1/4 tsp. hot sauce

Instructions

Sauté' chicken on high heat until brown in a large pot. Remove and set aside. Chop onions, celery, and green pepper and set aside.

Place oil and flour in pot. Stir well and brown to make a roux. When roux is done add chopped vegetables. Sauté on low heat for 10 minutes.

Slowly add chicken broth stirring constantly.

Add chicken and all other ingredients except the okra, shrimp and parsley, which will be saved for the end.

Cover and simmer on low for half an hour. Remove lid and cook for half an hour more, stirring occasionally.

Add shrimp, okra and parsley. Continue to cook on low heat uncovered for 15 minutes.

Chickpea Curry

Ingredients - Allergies: SF, GF, DF, EF, V, NF

- Curry Paste
- 2 cups cooked chickpeas
- 1/2 cup chopped cilantro

Instructions

Make Curry Paste. Mix in chickpeas and their liquid. Continue to cook and stir until all ingredients are well blended. Remove from heat. Stir in cilantro just before serving, reserving 1 tbsp. for garnish.

Red Curry Chicken

Ingredients - Allergies: SF, GF, DF, EF, NF

- 1 cup cubed chicken meat
- Curry Paste
- 2/3 cups tomato paste
- 2 Tbsp. coconut milk or cream
- Cilantro for garnishing

Instructions

Make Curry Paste. Add the tomato paste; stir and simmer until smooth. Add the chicken and the cream. Stir to combine. Simmer for 20 minutes. Serve with cilantro.

Braised Green Beans with Pork

Ingredients - Allergies: SF, GF, DF, EF, NF

- 2 cups fresh or frozen green beans
- 1 onion, finely chopped
- 2 cloves of garlic, thinly sliced
- 1/2 inch of peeled/sliced fresh ginger
- 1/2 tsp. red pepper flakes, or to taste
- 2 tomatoes, roughly chopped
- 2 tbsp. coconut oil
- 1 cup chicken broth
- Salt and ground black pepper
- 1/4 lemon, cut into wedges, to serve
- 10 oz. lean pork

Instructions

Cut each bean in half. Heat the coconut oil in a skillet over medium heat. Sauté the onion, garlic and ginger over medium heat until they are soft. Add the red pepper and tomatoes and sauté until the tomato begins to break down. Stir in the green beans. Add cubed lean pork. Add broth and bring to a simmer over medium heat. Cover and cook for so long that the beans get tender. Season to taste with salt and pepper. Serve with wedge of lemon on the side.

Ratatouille

Ingredients - Allergies: SF, GF, DF, EF, V, NF

- 1 large eggplants
- 2 small zucchinis
- 1 medium onions
- 1 red or green peppers
- 2 large tomatoes
- 1 cloves garlic, crushed
- 2 tbsp. coconut oil
- 1/2 tbsp. fresh basil
- Salt and freshly milled black pepper

Instructions

Cut eggplant and zucchini into 1 inch slices. Then cut each slice in half. Salt them and leave them for one hour. The salt will draw out the bitterness.

Chop peppers and onions. Skin the tomatoes by boiling them for few minutes. Then quarter them, take out the seeds and chop the flesh. Fry garlic and the onions in the coconut oil in a saucepan for a 10 minutes. Add the peppers. Dry the eggplant and zucchini and add them to the saucepan. Add the basil, salt and pepper. Stir and simmer for half an hour.

Add the tomato flesh, check the amount of seasoning and cook for an additional 15 minutes with the lid off.

Barbecued Beef

Ingredients - Allergies: SF, GF, DF, EF, NF

- 1/2 cups tomato paste
- 1 Tbsp. lemon juice
- 1/2 tbsp. mustard
- 1/8 tsp. salt
- 1 chopped carrot
- 1/8 tsp. ground black pepper
- 1/4 tsp. minced garlic
- 1 pound boneless chuck roast

Instructions

In a large bowl, combine tomato paste, lemon juice and mustard. Stir in salt, pepper and garlic.

Place chuck roast and carrot in a slow cooker. Pour tomato mixture over chuck roast. Cover, and cook on low for 7 to 9 hours. Remove chuck roast from slow cooker, shred with a fork, and return to the slow cooker. Stir meat to evenly coat with sauce. Continue cooking approximately 1 hour.

Beef Tenderloin with Roasted Shallots

Ingredients - Allergies: SF, GF, DF, EF

- 1/2 pound shallots, halved lengthwise and peeled
- 1/2 tbsp. olive oil or avocado oil
- salt and pepper to taste
- 1 cup beef broth
- 1/4 cup red wine
- 1/2 teaspoons tomato paste
- 1 pound beef tenderloin roast, trimmed
- 1/4 tsp. dried thyme
- 1 tbsp. coconut oil
- 1/2 tbsp. almond flour

Instructions

Heat oven to 375 degrees F. Toss shallots with olive oil to coat in a baking pan and season with salt and pepper. Roast until shallots are tender, stirring occasionally, about half an hour.
Combine wine and beef broth in a sauce pan and bring to a boil. Cook over high heat. Volume should be reduced by half. Add in tomato paste. Set aside.
Pat beef dry and sprinkle with salt and thyme and pepper. Add beef to pan oiled with coconut oil. Brown on all sides over high heat.
Put pan back to the oven. Roast beef about half an hour for medium rare. Transfer beef to platter. Cover loosely with foil.
Place pan on stove top and add broth mixture. Bring to boil and stir to scrape up any browned bits. Transfer to a different saucepan, and bring to simmer. Mix 1 1/2 tbsp. coconut oil and flour in small bowl and mix. Whisk into broth, and simmer until

sauce thickens. Stir in roasted shallots. Season with salt and pepper.

Cut beef into 1/2 inch thick slices. Spoon some sauce over.

Chili

Ingredients - Allergies: SF, GF, DF, EF, NF

- 1 tbsp. coconut oil
- 1 onion, chopped
- 1 cloves garlic, minced
- 1/4 pound ground beef
- 1/4 pound beef sirloin, cubed
- 1 cup diced tomatoes
- 1/4 cup strong brewed coffee
- 1/3 cup tomato paste
- 1 cups beef broth
- 1/4 tbsp. cumin seeds
- 1/4 tbsp. unsweetened cocoa powder
- 1/4 tsp. dried oregano
- 1/4 tsp. ground cayenne pepper
- 1/4 tsp. ground coriander
- 1/4 tsp. salt
- 1 1/2 cups cooked kidney beans
- 1 fresh hot chili peppers, chopped

Instructions

Heat oil in a saucepan over medium heat. Cook garlic, onions, sirloin and ground beef in oil until the meat is browned and the onions are translucent.
Mix in the diced tomatoes, coffee, tomato paste and beef broth. Season with oregano, cumin, cocoa powder, cayenne pepper, coriander and salt. Stir in hot chile peppers and 3 cups of the beans. Reduce heat to low, and simmer for two hours.

Stir in the 3 remaining cups of beans. Simmer for another 30 minutes.

Glazed Meatloaf

Ingredients - Allergies: SF, GF, DF, NF

- 1/4 cup tomato paste
- 1 Tbsp. lemon juice, divided
- 1/2 tsp. mustard powder
- 1 pounds ground beef
- 1/2 cup flax seeds meal
- 1/4 cup chopped onion
- 1 egg, beaten

Instructions

Heat oven to 350 degrees F. Combine mustard, tomato paste, 1/2 tbsp. lemon juice in a small bowl.

Combine onion, ground beef, flax, egg and remaining lemon juice in a separate larger bowl. And add 1/3 of the tomato paste mixture from the smaller bowl. Mix all well and place in a loaf pan.

Bake at 350 degrees F for one hour. Drain any excess fat and coat with remaining tomato paste mixture. Bake for 10 more minutes.

Eggplant Lasagna

Ingredients - Allergies: SF, GF, NF

- 1 large eggplant, peeled and sliced lengthwise into strips
- coconut oil
- salt and pepper

Meat Sauce

- 1/2 lbs ground sirloin or 1/2 lbs turkey breast
- 1 tbsp. coconut oil
- 1 onion, chopped
- 1 cloves chopped garlic
- 1/2 red pepper, chopped
- 8 ounce sliced mushrooms
- 1/2 tbsp. of oregano, basil and thyme each
- 1/2 tsp. fennel seed (optional)
- salt and pepper
- 1/2 tsp. red pepper flakes (optional)
- 1 cup chopped spinach
- 2 cups tomato sauce
- 1 cup diced tomatoes

Cheese Mixture

- 1 cup low-fat farmers cheese
- 1 egg
- 1 green onions, chopped

• 1/4 cup shredded low-fat mozzarella cheese (optional)

Instructions

Heat oven to 425 degrees.

Oil cookie sheet and arrange eggplant slice. Sprinkle with salt and pepper. Bake slices 5 minutes on each side. Lower oven temp to 375.

Brown onion, meat and garlic in coconut oil for 5 minutes. Add mushrooms and red pepper, and cook for 5 minutes. Add tomatoes, spinach and spices and simmer for 5-10 minutes.

Blend farmers' cheese, egg and onion mixture. Spread one third of meat sauce in bottom of a glass pan. Layer one half of eggplant slices and one half farmers' cheese. Repeat. Add last layer of sauce and then mozzarella on top.

Cover with foil. Bake at 375 degrees for one hour. Remove foil and bake until cheese is browned. Let it rest 10 minutes before serving.

Stuffed Eggplant

Serves – one half of eggplant per person

Allergies: SF, GF, DF, EF, NF

Rinse the eggplants. Cut off a slice from one end. Make a wide slit and salt them. Deseed tomatoes. Chop them finely. Cut the onions in thin slices. Chop the garlic cloves. Place them in a frying pan with coconut oil. Add the tomatoes, salt parsley, cumin, pepper, hot peppers and ground beef. Sauté for 10 minutes.

Squeeze eggplants, so the bitter juice goes out. Fill the wide slit with the ground beef mix. Pour the remaining mix over. Heat the oven to 375F in the meantime. Place eggplants a baking pan. Sprinkle them with olive oil, lemon juice and 1 cup of water. Cover the pan with a foil.

Stuffed Red Peppers with Beef

Ingredients - Allergies: SF, GF, DF, EF, NF

- 3 red bell peppers
- salt to taste
- 1/2 pound ground beef
- 1/4 cup chopped onion
- salt and pepper to taste
- 1 cup chopped tomatoes
- 1/4 cup uncooked brown rice or quinoa
- 1/4 cup water
- 1 cup tomato soup
- water as needed

Instructions

Bring a pot of salted water to a boil. Cut the tops off the peppers. Remove the seeds. Cook peppers in boiling water for 5 minutes and drain.
Sprinkle salt inside each pepper, and set aside.
In a skillet, sauté onions and beef until beef is browned. Drain off excess fat. Season with salt and pepper. Stir in rice, tomatoes and 1/2 cup water. Cover, and simmer until rice is tender. Remove from heat. Stir in the cheese.
Heat the oven to 350 degrees F. Stuff each pepper with the rice and beef mixture. Place peppers open side up in a baking dish. Combine tomato soup with just enough water to make the soup a gravy consistency in a separate bowl. Pour over the peppers.
Bake covered for 25 to 35 minutes.

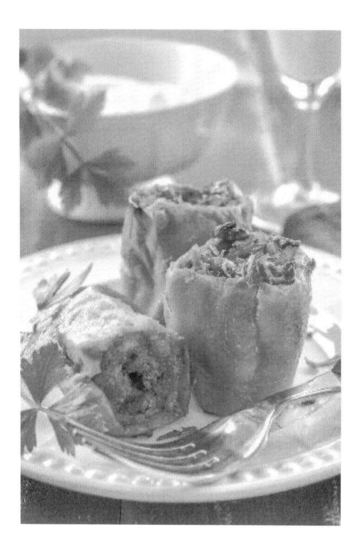

Superfoods Goulash

Ingredients - Allergies: SF, GF, DF, EF, NF

- 1 1/2 cups cauliflower
- 1/2 pound ground beef
- 1 small onion, chopped
- salt to taste
- ground black pepper to taste
- garlic to taste
- 1/2 cup cooked kidney beans
- 1/2 cup tomato paste

Brown the ground beef and onion in a skillet, over medium heat. Drain off the fat. Add garlic, salt and pepper to taste.
Stir in the cauliflower, kidney beans and tomato paste. Cook until cauliflower is done.

Frijoles Charros

Ingredients - Allergies: SF, GF, DF, EF, NF

- 1/2 pound dry pinto beans

- 1 clove garlic, chopped

- 1/2 tsp. salt

- 1/4 pound pork, diced

- 1/2 onion, chopped & 2 fresh tomatoes, diced

- few sliced sliced jalapeno peppers

- 1/4 cup chopped cilantro

Instructions

Place pinto beans in a slow cooker. Cover with water. Mix in garlic and salt. Cover, and cook 1 hour on High.

Cook the pork in a skillet over high heat until brown. Drain the fat. Place onion in the skillet. Cook until tender. Mix in jalapenos and tomatoes. Cook until heated through. Transfer to the slow cooker and stir into the beans. Continue cooking for 4 hours on Low. Mix in cilantro about half an hour before the end of the cook time.

Chicken Cacciatore

Ingredients - Allergies: SF, GF, DF, EF, NF

- 1 pound of chicken thighs, with skin on
- 1 Tbsp. extra virgin <u>olive</u> oil or <u>avocado</u> oil
- Salt
- 1 small sliced onion
- 1/4 cup red wine
- 1 sliced red or green bell pepper
- 2 ounces sliced cremini mushrooms
- 1 sliced garlic cloves
- 1 cup peeled and chopped tomatoes
- 1/2 tsp. ground black pepper
- 1/2 tsp. dry oregano
- 1/2 tsp. dry thyme
- 1/2 sprig fresh rosemary
- 1/2 tbsp. fresh parsley

Instructions

Pat the chicken on all sides with salt. Heat the olive oil in a skillet on medium. Brown few chicken pieces skin side down in the pan (don't overcrowd) for 5 minutes, then turn. Set aside. Make sure you have 1 tbsp. of the rendered fat left.

Add the onions, mushrooms and bell peppers to the pan. Increase the heat to medium high. Cook until the onions are tender, stirring, about 10 minutes. Add the garlic and cook a minute more.

Add the wine. Scrape up any browned bits and simmer until the wine is reduced by half. Add the tomatoes, pepper, oregano, thyme and a tsp. of salt. Simmer uncovered for maybe 5 more minutes. Put the chicken pieces on top of the tomatoes, skin side up. Lower the heat. Cover the skillet with the lid slightly ajar.

Cook the chicken on a low simmer. Turning and baste from time to time. Add rosemary and cook until the meat is tender, about 30 to 40 minutes. Garnish with parsley.

Cabbage Stewed with Meat

Ingredients - Allergies: SF, GF, DF, EF, NF

- 1 pound ground beef
- 1/2 cup beef stock
- 1 small chopped onion
- 1 bay leaf
- 1/8 tsp. pepper
- 1 sliced celery ribs
- 2 cups shredded cabbage
- 1 carrot, sliced
- 1/2 cup tomato paste
- 1/4 tsp. salt

Instructions

Brown ground meat in a pot. Add beef stock, onion, pepper and bay leaf. Cover and simmer until tender (approx.. 30 minutes). Add celery, cabbage and carrot.

Cover and simmer until vegetables are tender. Mix in tomato paste and seasoning blend. Simmer uncovered for 20 minutes.

Beef Stew with Peas and Carrots

Ingredients - Allergies: SF, GF, DF, EF, NF

- 1/2 cup chopped carrots
- 1/8 cup chopped onions
- 1 tbsp. coconut oil
- 1 cup green peas
- 1 cups beef stock
- 1/4 tsp. salt
- 1/8 tsp. ground black pepper
- 1/4 tsp. minced garlic
- 1 pound boneless chuck roast

Instructions

Cook the onions in coconut oil on medium until they are tender (few minutes). Add all other ingredients and stir. Cover and cook on low heat for 2 hours. Mix almond flour with some cold water, add to the stew and cook for another minute.

Green Chicken Stew

Ingredients - Allergies: SF, GF, DF, EF, NF

- 1 cups broccoli florets
- 1/4 cup chopped celery stalks
- 1/4 cup sliced leeks
- 1 tbsp. coconut oil
- 1/2 cups green peas
- 1 cups chicken stock
- 1/4 tsp. salt
- 1/8 tsp. ground black pepper
- 1/4 tsp. minced garlic
- 1 pounds boneless skinless chicken pieces

Instructions

Cook the leeks in coconut oil on medium until they are tender (few minutes). Add all other ingredients and stir. Cover and cook on low heat for 1 hour. Mix almond flour with some cold water, add to the stew and cook for another minute.

Irish Stew

Ingredients - Allergies: SF, GF, DF, EF, NF

- 1 small chopped onions
- 1 Tbsp. coconut oil
- 1 sprig dried thyme
- 1 pound chopped meat from lamb neck
- 2 chopped carrots
- 1 tbsp. brown rice
- 1 ½ cup chicken stock
- Salt
- Ground black pepper
- 1 bouquet garni (thyme, parsley and bay leaf)
- 1/2 bunch chopped parsley
- 1/2 bunch chives

Instructions

Cook the onions in coconut oil on medium until they are tender. Add the dried thyme and lamb and stir. Add brown rice, carrots and chicken stock. Add salt, pepper and bouquet garni. Cover and cook on low heat for 2 1/2 hours.

Garnish with parsley and chives.

Hungarian Pea Stew

Ingredients - Allergies: SF, GF, DF, EF, NF

- 1 & 1/2 cups green peas
- 1 pound cubed pork
- 1 tbsp <u>olive</u> oil or <u>avocado</u> oil
- 1 tbsp <u>almond</u> flour
- 1 tbsp chopped parsley
- 1/2 cup water
- 1/4 tsp salt
- 1/2 cup coconut milk
- 1/2 tsp coconut sugar

Instructions

Simmer the pork and green peas in the olive oil over medium heat until almost tender (approx. 10 minutes)

Add salt, chopped parsley, coconut sugar and almond flour, and cook for another minute.

Add water then milk and stir.

Cook for another 4 minutes over low heat, stirring occasionally.

Chicken Tikka Masala

Ingredients - Allergies: SF, GF, DF, EF, NF

- 1 pound chicken pieces, skinless, bone in
- 1 tbsp. toasted paprika
- 1 tbsp. toasted ground cumin
- 1/2 tsp. cayenne pepper
- 1 tbsp. toasted ground coriander seed
- 1 tsp. ground turmeric
- 3 chopped cloves garlic
- 1 tbsp. chopped fresh ginger
- 1/2 cups yogurt
- 1/4 cup lemon juice (4 to 6 lemons)
- 1/4 tsp. sea salt
- 1 tbsp. coconut oil
- 1/4 sliced onion
- 1 cups chopped tomatoes
- 1/4 cup chopped cilantro
- 1/4 cup coconut cream

Instructions

Score chicken deeply at 1-inch intervals with a knife. Place chicken in a large baking dish.

Combine coriander, cumin, paprika, turmeric, and cayenne in a bowl and mix. Set aside 3 tbsp. of this spice mixture. Combine remaining spice mixture with garlic garlic, yogurt, ginger, salt and lemon juice in a large bowl and combine. Pour marinade over chicken pieces and coat every surface (use hands). Refrigerate and marinate between 4 and 8 hours, turning occasionally.

Heat coconut oil in a large pot over medium-high heat and add remaining garlic and ginger. Add onions. Cook about 10 minutes, stirring occasionally. Add reserved spice mixture and cook until fragrant, about half a minute. Scrape up any browned bits from bottom of pan and add tomatoes and half of cilantro. Simmer for 15 minutes. Let cool slightly and puree.

Stir in coconut cream and remaining one quarter cup lemon juice. Season to taste with salt and set aside until chicken is cooked.

Cook chicken on a grill or under a broiler.

Remove chicken from bone and cut into rough bite-sized chunks. Add chicken chunks to pot of sauce. Bring to a simmer over medium heat and cook about 10 minutes.

Sprinkle with remaining cilantro.

Greek Beef Stew (Stifado)

Ingredients - Allergies: SF, GF, DF, EF, NF

- 2 pieces of veal or beef osso bucco
- 6 whole shallots, peeled
- 1 bay leaves
- 2 garlic cloves
- 3 sprigs rosemary
- 6 whole pimento
- 5 whole cloves
- 1/2 tsp ground nutmeg
- 1/2 cup olive oil or avocado oil
- 1/3 cup apple cider vinegar
- 1 tbsp. salt
- 2 cups tomato paste
- 1/4 tsp black pepper

Instructions

Mix vinegar and tomato paste and set aside. Place the meat, shallots, garlic and all spices in the pot.

Add the tomato paste, oil and vinegar. Cover the pot, bring to low boil and simmer on low for 2 hours. Do not open and stir, just shake the pot occasionally.

Meat Stew with Red Beans

Ingredients - Allergies: SF, GF, DF, EF, NF

- 1 tbsp. olive oil or avocado oil
- 1/4 chopped onion
- 1 pound lean cubed stewing beef
- 1 tsp. ground cumin
- 1 tsp. ground turmeric (optional)
- 1/4 tsp. ground cinnamon (optional)
- 1 cups water
- 1 tbsp. chopped fresh parsley
- 1 tbsp. snipped chives
- 1/2 cup cooked kidney beans
- 1/2 lemon, juice of
- 1/2 tbsp. almond flour
- salt and black pepper

Instructions

Sauté the onion in a pan with two tablespoons of the ive oil until tender.

Add beef and cook until meat is browned on all sides. Stir in turmeric, cinnamon (both optional) and cumin and cook for one minute. Add water and bring to a boil.

Cover and simmer over low heat for 45 minutes. Stir occasionally. Sauté parsley and chives with the remaining 1 tbsp. of olive oil for about 2 minutes and add this mixture to the beef. Add kidney beans and lemon juice and season with salt and pepper.

Stir in one tbsp. of almond flour mixed with a bit of water to thicken the stew. Simmer uncovered for half an hour until meat gets tender.

Beef, Parsnip, Celery Stew

Serves 2

Ingredients - Allergies: SF, GF, DF, EF, NF

- 1 pound cubed beef meat
- 1 chopped onion
- 2 chopped carrots
- 1 Tbsp. coconut oil
- 1/2 sprig dried thyme
- 1 chopped parsnip
- 1 tbsp. brown rice
- 1 cup beef stock
- Salt
- Ground black pepper
- 1 Tbsp. chopped parsley

Instructions

Put all ingredients in the slow cooker and cook on low for 8 hours.

Chicken Mushrooms & Olives Stew

Serves 2

Ingredients - Allergies: SF, GF, DF, EF, NF

- 1 pounds chicken with skin on
- 1 chopped carrot
- 1 small chopped onion
- 1 tbsp. coconut oil
- 1/2 cup sliced mushrooms
- 1/4 cup chopped celery
- 1/4 cup black olives
- 1/4 tsp. salt
- 1/8 tsp. ground black pepper
- 1/4 tsp. minced garlic
- 1/4 cup fresh parsley

Instructions

Put all ingredients in the crockpot, cover and cook on low 6 hours.

Chicken Pasanda Curry

Serves: 2

Ingredients - Allergies: SF, GF, DF, EF, NF

- 1 cup cubed chicken meat
- Curry Paste, but go low on the heat
- 1 cups tomato paste
- 1/4 cup coconut milk or cream
- Cilantro for garnishing

Instructions

Make Curry Paste. Add the tomato paste, chicken and the cream. Stir to combine, add to crockpot and cook on low for 3 hours.

Osso Bucco & Garlic Stew

Serves 2

Ingredients - Allergies: SF, GF, DF, EF, NF

- 2 cloves garlic
- 1 small chopped onion
- 1 chopped carrot
- 1 chopped celery stalk
- 1 tbsp. coconut oil
- 3/4 cup beef stock
- 1/4 tsp. salt
- 1/8 tsp. ground black pepper
- 1 tsp. chopped parsley
- 1 pound osso bucco

Instructions

Put all ingredients in the slow cooker and cook on low for 8 hours.

Beef Meatballs with White Beans

Serves 2

Ingredients - Allergies: SF, GF, DF, EF, NF

- 3/4 pounds baked meatballs (see recipe in bonus chapter)
- 1 Tbsp. coconut oil
- 1 cups uncooked white navy beans
- 1 1/2 cups beef stock
- Salt
- Ground black pepper
- 1 small chopped onion
- 1 Tbsp. chopped parsley
- 1 chopped carrot

Instructions

Add all ingredients but meatballs and cook on high for 4 hours. Add meatballs and cook on low for 2 hours more. Garnish with parsley.

Duck Stew

Serves 2

Ingredients - Allergies: SF, GF, DF, EF, NF

- 1 Tbsp. olive oil
- 1/2 pound chopped duck meat (1/2 inch wide)
- 1/4 pound duck liver, sliced
- 1 chopped carrot
- 1 celery stalk, chopped
- 1 small chopped onions
- 1 garlic cloves, chopped
- 1 cup chicken broth
- 1/2 cup sliced shiitake mushrooms
- 2 Tbsp. cup cilantro

Instructions

Put all ingredients in the slow cooker and cook on low for 4 Hrs.

Pork, Celery and Basil Stew

Serves 2

Ingredients - Allergies: SF, GF, DF, EF, NF

- 1 small chopped onion
- 1 Tbsp. coconut oil
- 1 pound chopped pork meat
- 1 chopped carrot
- 1 cup beef stock
- 1/4 cup red wine (optional)
- Salt
- Ground black pepper
- 1 Tbsp. chopped parsley
- 1 celery stalk, chopped
- 1 Tbsp. fresh basil

Instructions

Add all ingredients to slow cooker and cook on low for 8 hours.

Slow cooked Cabbage Rolls

Serves 2

Ingredients - Allergies: SF, GF, DF, EF, NF

1/2 pounds ground beef
1 small chopped onion
1 cup tomato sauce
1 pound cabbage or sauerkraut leaves
1/4 cup uncooked brown rice
1/4 tsp. salt
1/2 cup beef broth

Instructions

In a large mixing bowl combine onions, rice, flax, millet, ground walnuts and salt. Roll mixture into cabbage leaves and arrange them in a slow cooker dish. Pour broth and tomato sauce over rolls and cook on low for 6 hours.

Vegetarian Garbanzo Chili

Serves 2

Ingredients - Allergies: SF, GF, DF, EF, NF

- 1 chopped onion
- 1 Tbsp. coconut oil
- 1 large tomato, chopped
- 1/2 cup dry beans (kidney, black, pinto)
- 1/2 cup garbanzo beans
- 1 chopped carrot
- 1 chopped jalapeno peppers (watch for the heat)
- 1 + 1/2 cup beef stock
- Salt
- Ground black pepper
- 1 small bunch chopped spring onions

Instructions

Put all ingredients in the slow cooker and cook on low for 5 Hrs.

Red Peppers Pork Curry

Serves 2

Ingredients - Allergies: SF, GF, DF, EF, NF

- 1 cup sliced red peppers
- 3/4 cups chopped onions
- 1 tbsp. coconut oil
- 1/3 cup curry paste*
- 1 pound chopped pork meat

Instructions

Put ingredients in the slow cooker. Cover, and cook on low for 7 to 9 hours.

Beef Ratatouille

Serves 2

Ingredients - Allergies: SF, GF, DF, EF, NF

- 1/2 cup sliced zucchini
- 1/3 cup chopped onions
- 1 cup sliced eggplant
- 1/2 cups sliced red peppers (or tomato)
- 1 tbsp. coconut oil
- 1 tbsp. chopped garlic
- 1 tsp. salt and 1/2 tsp. ground pepper
- 1 pound cubed beef

Instructions

Put ingredients in the slow cooker. Cover, and cook on low for 7 to 9 hours.

Chicken, Green Peas and Red Peppers Stew
Serves 2

Ingredients - Allergies: SF, GF, DF, EF, NF

- 3/4 cups green peas
- 1/3 cup chopped onions
- 1/2 cups sliced red peppers
- 1 tbsp. coconut oil
- 1 cup chicken broth
- 1 tsp. salt and 1 tsp. ground pepper
- 1 pound cubed chicken

Instructions

Put ingredients in the slow cooker. Cover, and cook on low for 7 to 9 hours.

Crock Pot Turkey Roast Mediterranean style

Serves 2

Ingredients - Allergies: SF, GF, DF, EF, NF

- 1/4 cup Kalamata olives
- 1/4 cup chopped sun dried tomatoes
- 1/2 cup chicken broth
- 1 garlic clove, minced
- 3/4 cups chopped onions
- 1 tbsp. coconut oil
- 1 pound turkey breast
- Rub thyme, salt and ground black pepper.

Instructions

Put ingredients in the slow cooker. Cover, and cook on low for 7 to 9 hours.

Slow Cooker Pot Roast

Serves 2

Ingredients - Allergies: SF, GF, DF, EF, NF

- 1/3 cup sliced celery
- 1/2 cup chopped carrot
- 1 cup beef broth
- 1/4 cup red wine (optional) & 3 garlic cloves (optional)
- 1/3 cup chopped onions
- 1 tbsp. coconut oil
- 1 pounds beef chuck roast
- Rub thyme, salt and ground black pepper. Add 1 bay leaf.

Instructions

Put ingredients in the slow cooker. Cover, and cook on low for 7 to 9 hours.

Beef, Leeks & Mushrooms Stew

Serves 2

Ingredients - Allergies: SF, GF, DF, EF, NF

- 3/4 cups chopped carrots
- 1/2 cup chopped onions
- 1 tbsp. coconut oil
- 1/2 cup chopped leeks
- Salt & ground black pepper to taste
- 1 cup sliced mushrooms
- 1/2 cup sliced tomatoes
- 1 pound beef meat cut into stripes

Instructions

Put ingredients in the slow cooker. Cover, and cook on low for 7 to 9 hours.

Chicken, Garlic & Tomato Stew

Serves 2

Ingredients - Allergies: SF, GF, DF, EF, NF

- 1 cup tomatoes
- 3/4 cup chopped onions
- 1 tbsp. coconut oil
- 1 small garlic bulb, cut across
- Salt, ground black pepper and ground cumin to taste
- 1/4 Tbsp. minced garlic
- 1 pound chicken breast meat cut into stripes

Instructions

Put ingredients in the slow cooker. Cover, and cook on low for 7 to 9 hours.

Minced Pork, Tomato & Red Peppers Stew

Serves 2

Ingredients - Allergies: SF, GF, DF, EF, NF

- 1 cup quartered tomatoes
- 1/4 cup chopped onions
- 1 tbsp. coconut oil
- 3/4 cup chopped red peppers
- Salt, ground black pepper and ground cumin to taste
- 1/2 cup shredded carrots
- 1 pound minced pork meat

Instructions

Put ingredients in the slow cooker. Cover, and cook on low for 7 to 9 hours.

Beef, Eggplant, Celery & Peppers Stew
Serves 2

Ingredients - Allergies: SF, GF, DF, EF, NF

- 1/2 cup cubed eggplant
- 1 cup chopped onions
- 1 tbsp. coconut oil
- 1/3 cup sliced celery
- Salt, ground black pepper to taste
- 1/2 cup sliced red peppers
- 1 pound beef meat cut into stripes

Instructions

Put ingredients in the slow cooker. Cover, and cook on low for 7 to 9 hours.

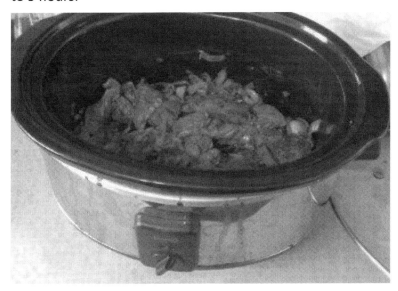

Chicken & Onion Stew

Serves 2

Ingredients - Allergies: SF, GF, DF, EF, NF

- 1/2 cup sliced mushrooms
- 2 large onions, quartered
- 1 tbsp. coconut oil
- Salt, ground black pepper to taste
- 3/4 cup chicken stock
- 1 pound chicken drumsticks with skin on

Instructions

Put ingredients in the slow cooker. Cover, and cook on low for 7 to 9 hours.

Leeks, Mushrooms & Pork Neck Meat

Serves 2

Ingredients - Allergies: SF, GF, DF, EF, NF

- 1 cup mushrooms, sliced
- 3/4 cup chopped leeks
- 1 tbsp. coconut oil
- Salt, ground black pepper and ground cumin to taste
- 1 bay leaves & 1 Tbsp. chopped garlic
- 1 cup beef stock
- 1 Tbsp. sesame seeds
- 1 Tbsp. cup chopped spring onions
- 1 pound pork neck meat

Instructions

Put all ingredients in the slow cooker except spring onions and sesame seeds. Cover, and cook on low for 9 hours. Sprinkle with chopped spring onions and sesame seeds.

Broccoli, Pork & Peppers

Serves 2

Ingredients - Allergies: SF, GF, DF, EF, NF

- 1/2 cup sliced yellow and orange peppers
- 1/4 cup chopped onions
- 1 tbsp. coconut oil
- Salt, ground black pepper to taste
- 1/2 cup beef stock
- 1/2 pound pork chops
- 1/2 pounds pork neck
- 1 Tbsp. minced garlic.
- 1 cup broccoli florets

Instructions

Put ingredients in the slow cooker. Cover, and cook on low for 8 hours.

Haitian Chicken Broccoli

Serves 2

Ingredients - Allergies: SF, GF, DF, EF, NF

- 1 cup broccoli florets
- 1/2 cup chopped onions
- 1 tbsp. coconut oil
- Salt, ground black pepper to taste
- 1 cup chicken stock
- 1 pound cubed chicken meat
- 1/4 tsp. dried red pepper flakes (to taste).
- 1 whole clove (discard after cooking)
- 1 Tsp. minced garlic
- 1 Tsp. apple vinegar

Instructions

Put ingredients in the slow cooker. Cover, and cook on low for 8 hours.

Leeks, Cauliflower, Chicken & Carrot

Serves 2

Ingredients - Allergies: SF, GF, DF, EF, NF

- 1 cup sliced leeks
- 1/2 cup carrot
- 1 tbsp. coconut oil
- Salt, ground black pepper to taste
- 1 cup chicken stock
- 1 pound cubed chicken meat
- 1 Tsp. minced ginger & 1 Tsp. minced garlic.
- 1 stick celery, chopped

Instructions

Put ingredients in the slow cooker. Cover, and cook on low for 8 hours.

Okra & Pork Stew

Serves 2

Ingredients - Allergies: SF, GF, DF, EF, NF

- 1 cup sliced okra
- 1/2 cup chopped onions
- 1 tbsp. coconut oil
- Salt, ground black pepper to taste
- 1 cup beef stock
- 1 pound pork neck meat
- 2 cloves garlic, halved lengthwise
- 1 stick celery, chopped

Instructions

Put ingredients in the slow cooker. Cover, and cook on low for 8 hours.

Chicken, Black Beans and Cauliflower

Serves 2

Ingredients - Allergies: SF, GF, DF, EF, NF

- 1 cup cauliflower
- 1/4 cup black beans
- 1 cup chopped onions & 1 carrot - chopped
- 1 tbsp. coconut oil
- Salt, ground black pepper to taste
- 1 cup chicken stock
- 1 pound dark chicken meat
- 1 Tsp. minced garlic & 1/4 tsp. ground cumin

Instructions

Put ingredients in the slow cooker. Cover, and cook on low for 8 hours.

Celery, Carrots & Cauliflower Pork
Serves 2

Ingredients - Allergies: SF, GF, DF, EF, NF

- 1 cup sliced celery
- 1/2 cup chopped onions
- 1 tbsp. coconut oil
- Salt, ground black pepper to taste
- 1 cup beef stock
- 1 pound cubed pork meat
- 1 cup chopped carrots
- 1 cup chopped cauliflower
- 1 Tsp. minced garlic & 1 bay leaf (discard after cooking).

Instructions

Put ingredients in the slow cooker. Cover, and cook on low for 8 hours.

Slow Cooked Carnitas

Serves 2

Ingredients - Allergies: SF, GF, DF, EF, NF

- 1 cup chopped onions
- 1 tbsp. coconut oil
- Salt, ground black pepper to taste
- 1/2 pounds pork shoulder
- 1/2 pounds pork neck
- 1/4 Jalapeno pepper, chopped (to taste).
- 1 Tsp. minced garlic.
- 1/2 Tsp. ground cumin.

Instructions

Put ingredients in the slow cooker. Cover, and cook on low for 8 hours.

Chicken Green Curry

Serves 2

Ingredients - Allergies: SF, GF, DF, EF, NF

- 1/4 cup chopped onions
- 1/4 cup coconut milk
- 1/2 lime - juice & 1/2 cup chicken broth
- 1/4 cup chopped cilantro & 1 clove garlic.
- 1 pound chicken meat
- 1 cup sliced veggies (green beans and green peppers)
- 1 Tbsp. curry paste
- 1 Tbsp. fish sauce

Instructions

Blend lime, onions, curry paste, cilantro and spices. Put chicken and other ingredients in the slow cooker and pour blended ingredients over. Cover, and cook on low for 8 hours. Decorate with fresh basil leaves.

Two Beans Chili

Serves 2

Ingredients - Allergies: SF, GF, DF, EF, NF

- 1 tbsp. coconut oil
- 1 small onion, chopped
- 1 clove garlic, minced
- 1/2 pound ground beef
- 1/2 pound beef sirloin, cubed
- 1 cup diced tomatoes
- 1/4 cup strong brewed coffee
- 1/4 cup tomato paste
- 1/2 cups beef broth
- 1 tsp. cumin seeds
- 1/4 tsp. dried oregano
- 1/4 tsp. ground cayenne pepper
- 1/4 tsp. ground coriander
- 1/4 tsp. salt
- 1 cup cooked kidney beans
- 1/2 cup cooked navy beans
- 1 fresh hot chili peppers, chopped

Instructions

Put ingredients in the slow cooker. Cover, and cook on low for 4 hours.

Chicken & Artichoke Hearts

Serves 2

Ingredients - Allergies: SF, GF, DF, EF, NF

- 1/2 cup chopped onions
- 1 tbsp. coconut oil
- Salt, ground black pepper to taste
- 1 pounds chicken meat
- 1 cup chopped carrots.
- 2 Artichokes, tops sliced, trimmed
- 1 Tsp. ground cumin.
- 1/2 cup chicken broth

Instructions

Put ingredients in the slow cooker. Cover, and cook on low for 8 hours.

Green Peppers, Chicken and Green Onions
Serves 2

Ingredients - Allergies: SF, GF, DF, EF, NF

- 1/2 cups chopped green onions
- 1 tbsp. coconut oil
- Salt, ground black pepper to taste
- 1 pound chopped chicken meat
- 1/2 cups sliced green peppers
- 1 Tsp. minced garlic.
- 1/4 Tbsp. ground cumin.

Instructions

Put ingredients in the slow cooker. Cover, and cook on low for 8 hours.

Black Bean Chicken Chili

Serves 2

Ingredients - Allergies: SF, GF, DF, EF, NF

- 1 tbsp. coconut oil
- 1/2 onions, chopped
- 1 clove garlic, minced
- 1/2 pounds cubed chicken meat
- 1/2 cups diced red and yellow peppers
- 1/2 cups sliced celery
- 1/4 cup tomato paste
- 1/2 cups chicken broth
- 1/2 tsp. cumin seeds
- 1/4 tsp. dried oregano
- 1/4 tsp. ground cayenne pepper
- 1/4 tsp. ground coriander
- 1/4 tsp. salt
- 1/2 cups black beans
- 1 fresh hot chili pepper, chopped

Instructions

Put ingredients in the slow cooker. Cover, and cook on low for 8 hours.

Haitian Spinach Shrimp Stew
Serves 2

Ingredients - Allergies: SF, GF, DF, EF, NF

- 1/2 cups chopped onions
- 1 tbsp. coconut oil
- Salt, ground black pepper to taste
- 1 pound shrimp
- 1 cup spinach leaves
- 1/4 tsp. dried red pepper flakes (to taste).
- 1 whole clove (discard after cooking)
- 1/2 cups fish broth
- 1/4 cup tomato paste.
- 1/4 lime – juice only & a pinch ground cloves

Instructions

Put ingredients in the slow cooker. Cover, and cook on low for 8 hours.

Cabbage & Pork Stew

Serves 2

Ingredients - Allergies: SF, GF, DF, EF, NF

- 1/2 cups chopped onions
- 1 tbsp. coconut oil
- Salt, ground black pepper to taste
- 1/2 pounds pork shoulder
- 1/2 pounds pork neck
- 1 cup shredded cabbage
- 1 Tsp. minced garlic.
- 1/4 Tsp. ground cumin.

Instructions

Put ingredients in the slow cooker. Cover, and cook on low for 8 hours.

Parihuela – Peruvian Seafood Stew
Serves 2

Ingredients - Allergies: SF, GF, DF, EF, NF

- 1/2 pound cod filet & 1/4 pound seabass

- 2 Tbsp. olive oil

- 1 squid, cut into rings

- 1/4 cup thinly sliced onions

- 1 cloves garlic, crushed

- 1 small tomato, chopped

- 1/2 sweet red pepper, chopped

- 1 stalk celery, thinly sliced

- 1 sprigs fresh thyme or 1/4 tsp. dried thyme

- 1 bay leaf

- 1 whole clove

- 1 Tsp. grated ginger

- 1/4 lime - juice

- 1/2 teaspoon salt

- 1/4 tsp. ground black pepper

- 1/2 cup clam juice or fish broth

- 1/4 cup white wine

Instructions

Instructions

Put ingredients in the slow cooker. Cover, and cook on low for 4 hours.

Seafood & Mushrooms Stew
Serves 2

Ingredients - Allergies: SF, GF, DF, EF, NF

- 1/2 pound seabass

- 1 Tbsp. olive oil

- 1/4 cup shrimp

- 1 squid, cut into rings

- 1/4 cup thinly sliced onions

- 1 cloves garlic, crushed

- 1/4 cup sliced carrots

- 1/2 cup sliced Portobello mushrooms

- 1 Tsp. grated ginger

- 1/4 lime - juice

- 1/2 teaspoons salt

- 1/4 tsp. ground black pepper

- 1/2 cups fish broth

- 1/4 cup white wine

Instructions

Put ingredients in the slow cooker. Cover, and cook on low for 4 hours.

Duck Curry

Serves 2

Ingredients - Allergies: SF, GF, DF, EF, NF

- 1/2 cups chopped onions
- 1/4 cup chopped carrots
- 1/4 cup chopped zucchini
- 1 tbsp. coconut oil
- 1 pound. duck meat
- 1 Tbsp. Curry Paste, but go low on the heat
- 1/2 cups tomato paste
- 1/4 cup coconut milk or cream
- Cilantro for garnishing

Instructions

Make Curry Paste. Add the tomato paste, chicken, veggies and the cream. Stir to combine, add to crockpot and cook on low for 8 hours.

Eggplant Red Pepper Stew
Serves 2

Ingredients - Allergies: SF, GF, DF, EF, NF

- 1/2 cup chopped onions
- 1 tbsp. coconut oil
- Salt, ground black pepper to taste
- 1 pound cubed eggplant
- 1 cup sliced red peppers
- 1/4 tsp. dried red pepper flakes (to taste).
- 1/4 cup tomato paste.

Instructions

Put ingredients in the slow cooker. Cover, and cook on low for 8 hours.

Shrimp, Onion & Cilantro Stew

Serves 2

Ingredients - Allergies: SF, GF, DF, EF, NF

- 1 cups quartered onions
- 1 tbsp. coconut oil
- Salt, ground black pepper to taste
- 1 pound shrimp
- 1/4 tsp. dried red pepper flakes (to taste).
- 1/4 cup cilantro
- 1/2 cups fish broth
- 1/4 cup tomato paste.

Instructions

Put ingredients in the slow cooker. Cover, and cook on low for 8 hours.

Venison Green Beans Onion Stew

Serves 2

Ingredients - Allergies: SF, GF, DF, EF, NF

- 1 cup quartered onions
- 1 tbsp. coconut oil
- Salt, ground black pepper to taste
- 1 pounds venison meat
- 1/4 tsp. dried red pepper flakes (to taste).
- 1 whole clove (discard after cooking)
- 1 cup beef broth
- 1/2 cup green beans

Instructions

Put ingredients in the slow cooker. Cover, and cook on low for 8 hours.

Pork Cauliflower Stew

Serves 2

Ingredients - Allergies: SF, GF, DF, EF, NF

- 1/2 cup chopped onions
- 2 tbsp. coconut oil
- Salt, ground black pepper to taste
- 1 pound pork neck meat
- 1/2 cup sliced green onions
- 1/2 cup chopped carrots
- 3/4 cup beef broth
- 1 cup cauliflower
- 1/2 cup sliced tomatoes

Instructions

Put ingredients in the slow cooker. Cover, and cook on low for 8 hours. Sprinkle with sliced green onions.

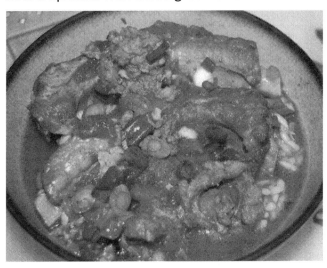

Sweet Potato Veal Stew

Serves 2

Ingredients - Allergies: SF, GF, DF, EF, NF

- 1/2 cups chopped onions
- 2 tbsp. coconut oil
- Salt, ground black pepper to taste
- 1 pounds veal neck meat
- 1 cup chopped sweet potato
- 1/2 cups beef broth

Instructions

Put ingredients in the slow cooker. Cover, and cook on low for 8 hours.

Pork Broccoli Carrot Stew

Serves 2

Ingredients - Allergies: SF, GF, DF, EF, NF

- 1/2 cups chopped onions
- 2 tbsp. coconut oil
- Salt, ground black pepper to taste
- 1 pounds cubed pork meat
- 1 cup broccoli
- 1 cup beef broth
- 1/2 cup sliced carrots

Instructions

Put ingredients in the slow cooker. Cover, and cook on low for 8 hours.

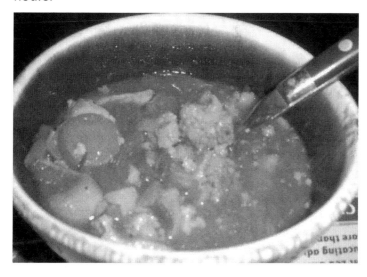

Moroccan Lamb & Mushrooms Stew

Serves 2

Ingredients - Allergies: SF, GF, DF, EF, NF

- 1/2 cups chopped onions
- 2 tbsp. coconut oil
- Salt, ground black pepper to taste
- 1 pound lamb neck meat
- 1/4 tsp. each: cumin, coriander, fennel seeds
- 1/4 tsp. dried red pepper flakes (to taste).
- 1/4 cup dried apricots
- 1/2 cup beef broth
- 1/4 cup tomato paste.
- 1/2 cups whole mushrooms
- 1/4 cup cilantro

Instructions

Put ingredients in the slow cooker. Cover, and cook on low for 8 hours. Sprinkle with cilantro.

Shrimp Peppers Stew

Serves 2

Ingredients - Allergies: SF, GF, DF, EF, NF

- 1/2 cups chopped onions
- 2 tbsp. coconut oil
- Salt, ground black pepper to taste
- 1 pound shrimp
- 1/4 tsp. dried red pepper flakes (to taste).
- 1 cup sliced red peppers
- 1/2 cup tomato paste.

Instructions

Put ingredients in the slow cooker. Cover, and cook on low for 8 hours.

Afghan Stew

Serves 2

Ingredients - Allergies: SF, GF, DF, EF, NF

- 1/2 cups chopped onions & 2 minced garlic cloves
- 2 tbsp. coconut oil
- Salt, ground black pepper to taste
- 1 pound chicken thighs
- 1/4 tsp. dried red pepper flakes (to taste).
- 1/4 tsp. cinnamon & 1 tsp. turmeric.
- 1/4 tsp. ground cardamom.
- 1/2 tbsp. parsley for decoration.
- 1 cup whole green peppers
- 1/2 cup beef broth & 1 cup tomato paste

Instructions

Put ingredients in the slow cooker. Cover, and cook on low for 8 hours. Decorate with parsley.

Chicken, Capers, Olives, Anchovy & Zucchini Stew

Serves 2

Ingredients - Allergies: SF, GF, DF, EF, NF

- 1/2 cups chopped onions
- 2 tbsp. coconut oil
- Salt, ground black pepper to taste
- 1 pound cubed chicken
- 1/4 cup olives.
- 1 Tsp. capers & 1 Tsp. anchovy
- 1 cup sliced zucchini
- 1/2 cup tomato paste.

Instructions

Put ingredients in the slow cooker. Cover, and cook on low for 8 hours.

Hunter's Green Beans Chicken Stew

Serves 2

Ingredients - Allergies: SF, GF, DF, EF, NF

- 1/2 cups chopped onions & 2 minced garlic cloves
- 2 tbsp. coconut oil
- Salt, ground black pepper to taste
- 1 pound chicken thighs
- 1/4 tsp. dried red pepper flakes (to taste).
- 1/2 cup mushrooms & 1 bay leaf
- 1/2 cup chopped tomatoes & 1 Tsp. fresh rosemary
- 1 cup green beans cut in 2 inch pieces
- 2 cups chicken broth & 1 cup white wine

Instructions

Put ingredients in the slow cooker. Cover, and cook on low for 8 hours.

Kale Chicken Jambalaya

Serves 2

Ingredients - Allergies: SF, GF, DF, EF, NF

- 1 cup chopped onions & 2 minced garlic cloves
- 2 tbsp. coconut oil & 1 tsp. turmeric
- Salt, ground black pepper to taste
- 3/4 pound cubed chicken & 1/4 pound shrimp
- 1/4 tsp. dried red pepper flakes (to taste).
- 1 cup kale & 1/2 cup mushrooms
- 1/4 cup tomato paste & 1/2 cup chicken broth
- 1/4 cup corn & 1/4 cup chopped carrot

Instructions

Put ingredients in the slow cooker. Cover, and cook on low for 8 hours.

Minced Pork and Veal Stew

Serves 2

Ingredients - Allergies: SF, GF, DF, EF, NF

- 1/2 cups finely chopped onions
- 2 tbsp. coconut oil
- Salt, ground black pepper to taste
- 1/2 pound minced pork and veal each
- 1 clove garlic, minced
- 1 cup finely chopped celery
- 1 cups finely chopped carrot
- 1/2 cup beef broth

Instructions

Put ingredients in the slow cooker. Cover, and cook on low for 8 hours.

Olives & Chicken Stew

Serves 2

Ingredients - Allergies: SF, GF, DF, EF, NF

- 1 cup chopped onions
- 2 tbsp. coconut oil
- Salt, ground black pepper to taste
- 1 pound chicken thighs
- 1/4 tsp. dried red pepper flakes (to taste).
- 1/2 cup sliced olives
- 1 cup tomato paste.

Instructions

Put ingredients in the slow cooker. Cover, and cook on low for 8 hours.

Pulled Pork

Serves 2

Ingredients - Allergies: SF, GF, DF, EF, NF

- 1 cup chopped onions & 2 minced garlic cloves
- 2 tbsp. coconut oil
- Salt, ground black pepper to taste
- 1 pound pork shoulder
- 1/4 tsp. dried red pepper flakes (to taste).
- 1/4 cup chicken broth & 1 Tbsp. apple cider vinegar
- 1/4 cup tomato paste & 1/2 tsp. ground cumin
- 1 tsp. mustard powder

Instructions

Put ingredients in the slow cooker. Cover, and cook on low for 8 hours.

Chicken, Olives, Capers & Eggplant Stew

Serves 2

Ingredients - Allergies: SF, GF, DF, EF, NF

- 1 cup chopped onions
- 2 tbsp. coconut oil
- Salt, ground black pepper to taste
- 1 pound cubed chicken
- 1/4 cup olives & 1Tbsp. capers
- 1/2 cup cauliflower florets
- 1 cup sliced eggplant
- 1/4 cup tomato paste.

Instructions

Put ingredients in the slow cooker. Cover, and cook on low for 8 hours.

Turkish Chicken Stew

Serves 2

Ingredients - Allergies: SF, GF, DF, EF, NF

- 1 cup chopped onions & 1 minced garlic clove
- 2 tbsp. coconut oil
- Salt, ground black pepper to taste
- 1 pound chicken thighs
- 1/4 tsp. dried red pepper flakes (to taste).
- 1 cup sliced red peppers
- 1 cup sliced eggplant or zucchini
- 1/4 cup tomato paste. & 1/4 cups brown rice
- 1/4 tsp. ground cumin & 1 star anise (discard before serving)

Instructions

Put ingredients in the slow cooker. Cover, and cook on low for 8 hours.

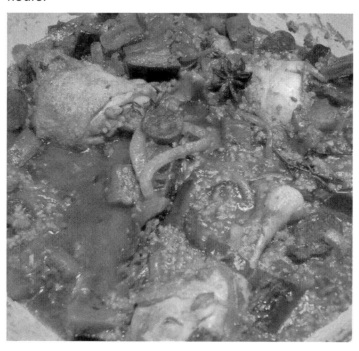

Veal & Red Peppers Stew

Serves 2

Ingredients - Allergies: SF, GF, DF, EF, NF

- 1 cup chopped onions & 2 minced garlic cloves
- 2 tbsp. coconut oil
- Salt, ground black pepper to taste
- 1 pound cubed veal
- 1/4 tsp. dried red pepper flakes (to taste).
- 1 cup sliced red peppers
- 1/2 cup tomato paste.

Instructions

Put ingredients in the slow cooker. Cover, and cook on low for 8 hours.

Chinese Eggplant, Chicken & Green Onions Stew

Serves 2

Ingredients - Allergies: SF, GF, DF, EF, NF

- 1 cup chopped onions
- 2 tbsp. coconut oil
- Salt, ground black pepper to taste
- 1 pound cubed chicken
- 1/4 cup sliced green onions
- 1 cup chicken broth
- 1 cup halved Chinese eggplants
- 1/4 cup tomato paste.

Instructions

Put ingredients in the slow cooker. Cover, and cook on low for 8 hours.

Pumpkin, Chicken, & Chinese Celery Stew

Serves 2

Ingredients - Allergies: SF, GF, DF, EF, NF

- 1 cup chopped onions
- 2 tbsp. coconut oil
- Salt, ground black pepper to taste
- 1 pound dark chicken meat
- 1/4 cup Chinese Celery
- 1/4 cup green peas & 1/4 cup sliced carrots
- 1 cup sliced pumpkin
- 1/2 cup chicken broth

Instructions

Put ingredients in the slow cooker. Cover, and cook on low for 8 hours.

Spicy Shrimp & Eggplant Stew

Serves 2

Ingredients - Allergies: SF, GF, DF, EF, NF

- 1 cups chopped onions
- 2 tbsp. coconut oil
- Salt, ground black pepper to taste
- 1 pounds shrimp
- 1/4 cup sliced celery
- 1 Tbsp. chopped parsley
- 1 cup sliced eggplant
- 1/2 cup tomato paste

Instructions

Put ingredients in the slow cooker. Cover, and cook on low for 8 hours.

Veal, Tomato, Garlic, Corn & Zucchini Stew

Serves 2

Ingredients - Allergies: SF, GF, DF, EF, NF

- 1 cup chopped onions
- 2 tbsp. coconut oil
- Salt, ground black pepper to taste
- 1 pound cubed veal
- 1/4 cup corn
- 3 cloves garlic
- 1 cup sliced zucchini
- 1 cup sliced tomatoes.

Instructions

Put ingredients in the slow cooker. Cover, and cook on low for 8 hours.

Chicken, Chickpeas, Tomato, Peppers & Eggplant Stew

Serves 2

Ingredients - Allergies: SF, GF, DF, EF, NF

- 1 cups chopped onions
- 2 tbsp. coconut oil
- Salt, ground black pepper to taste
- 1 pound cubed chicken
- 1/4 cup chickpeas
- 1/2 cup sliced peppers
- 1 cup sliced eggplant
- 1/4 cup sliced tomatoes

Instructions

Put ingredients in the slow cooker. Cover, and cook on low for 8 hours.

Mixed Seafood, Saffron & Sundried Tomatoes

Serves 2

Ingredients - Allergies: SF, GF, DF, EF, NF

- 1 cup sundried tomatoes
- 2 cups chopped onions
- 2 tbsp. coconut oil
- 1/4 cup olive oil mixed with 1 tsp. saffron
- Salt
- 2 cups white wine
- 4 pounds frozen mixed seafood

Instructions

Put ingredients in the slow cooker. Cover, and cook on high for 90 minutes.

Chicken and Sweet Potato

Serves 2

Ingredients - Allergies: SF, GF, DF, EF, NF

- 2 cups cubed sweet potato
- 2 cups chopped onions
- 2 tbsp. coconut oil
- 3 red peppers, chopped
- Salt, ground black pepper and ground cumin to taste
- 2 cups chicken stock
- 4 pounds chicken meat

Instructions

Put ingredients in the slow cooker. Cover, and cook on low for 7 to 9 hours.

Black Bean Cuban Stew

Serves 2

Ingredients - Allergies: SF, GF, DF, EF, NF

- 1/2 cup sliced carrot
- 1/2 cup chopped onions
- 1 small red pepper, chopped
- Salt, 1 Tsp. ground cayenne pepper and 1 Tbsp. cumin seeds
- 2 Tbsp. corn
- 3/4 cup dry black beans
- 2 Tbsp. tomato paste
- 3/4 cup beef broth
- 1/4 tsp. ground coriander
- 1 pound pork neck meat, cubed

Instructions

Put ingredients in the slow cooker. Cover, and cook on low for 7 to 9 hours.

Chicken and Garbanzo Stew

Serves 2

Ingredients - Allergies: SF, GF, DF, EF, NF

- 1/2 cup dry garbanzo beans
- 1/2 cups chopped onions
- 1 tbsp. coconut oil
- 3/4 cup tomatoes, chopped
- 1/4 cup chopped carrot
- 1/4 cup sliced celery
- 1 garlic clove, minced
- Salt, ground black pepper and ground cumin to taste
- 3/4 cups chicken stock
- 1 pound chicken meat

Instructions

Put ingredients in the slow cooker. Cover, and cook on low for 7 to 9 hours.

Spicy Beef Stew – Yukgaejang (Korean Recipe)
Serves 2

Ingredients - Allergies: SF, GF, DF, EF, NF

- 1/2 cups dried shiitake mushrooms
- 1/4 cup chopped onions
- 1 clove minced garlic
- 1/2 Tsp. minced ginger
- 1/2 cups green onions, cut in half
- 1 tsp. sesame oil
- 1/2 cups sprouts
- 2 Tsp. Fish sauce, hot pepper flakes to taste
- 1/2 cups chicken stock
- 1 pound beef brisket

Instructions

Put ingredients in the slow cooker. Cover, and cook on low for 7 to 9 hours.

Kale, Quinoa and Beans Stew

Serves 2

Ingredients - Allergies: SF, GF, DF, EF, NF

- 3/4 cup raw kidney beans
- 1/2 cup chopped onions
- 1/2 cup chopped kale
- 1/4 cup sliced carrot
- 1 tbsp. coconut oil
- 1/2 cup tomatoes, chopped
- Salt, ground black pepper and ground cumin to taste
- 1 cup chicken or vegetable stock
- 1 Tbsp. quinoa

Instructions

Put ingredients in the slow cooker. Cover, and cook on low for 7 to 9 hours.

Veal & Sweet Potato Stew

Serves 2

Ingredients - Allergies: SF, GF, DF, EF, NF

- 1/2 cup cubed sweet potato
- 1/2 cups chopped onions
- 1/4 cup chopped carrots
- 1/2 cup chopped celery
- 1 tbsp. coconut oil
- 1 small red pepper, chopped
- 2 Tbsp. tomato paste
- Salt, ground black pepper and ground cumin to taste
- 3/4 cup beef stock
- 1 pound veal meat

Instructions

Put ingredients in the slow cooker. Cover, and cook on low for 7 to 9 hours.

Teriyaki Chicken & Carrots

Serves 2

Ingredients - Allergies: SF, GF, DF, EF, NF

- 1/2 cup sliced carrots
- 1 Tsp. minced ginger & 1 garlic clove, minced
- 1 Tsp. honey
- 1 Tbsp. rice or apple cider vinegar
- 1 tbsp. coconut oil
- 1/4 cup onions, chopped
- 1 Tbsp. fish sauce
- 1/2 cup chicken stock & 1 Tbsp. cornstarch (optional)
- 1 pound chicken meat

Instructions

Put ingredients in the slow cooker. Cover, and cook on low for 7 to 9 hours.

Spicy Garbanzo and Spinach Stew

Serves 2

Ingredients - Allergies: SF, GF, DF, EF, NF

- 1/2 cups dry garbanzo beans
- 3/4 cups chopped onions
- 1 cup spinach
- 1 tbsp. coconut oil
- 1 red pepper, chopped
- 1/4 cup tomato paste
- Salt, ground cayenne pepper and ground cumin to taste
- 3/4 cup chicken stock
- 1 pound chicken meat

Instructions

Put ingredients in the slow cooker. Cover, and cook on low for 7 to 9 hours.

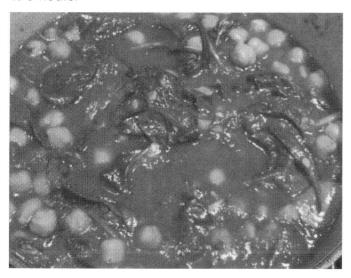

Cacciucco - Shrimp, Mussels, Fish & Scallops Stew

Serves 2

Ingredients - Allergies: SF, GF, DF, EF, NF

- 1/2 cup tomato paste
- 1/2 cups chopped onions
- 1 tbsp. coconut oil
- 1/4 cup cherry tomatoes
- Salt, 1 Tbsp. chopped dill.
- 1 cup fish or vegetable stock
- 1/4 pound shrimp
- 1/4 pound mussels
- 1/4 pound scallops
- 1/4 pound local fish

Instructions

Put ingredients in the slow cooker. Cover, and cook on low for 7 to 9 hours.

Lamb and Peppers Stew

Serves 2

Ingredients - Allergies: SF, GF, DF, EF, NF

- 1/2 cups chopped onions
- 1 tbsp. coconut oil
- 1 red pepper, chopped
- 1 yellow pepper, chopped
- Salt, ground black pepper and ground cumin to taste
- 1/2 cup beef stock
- 1/4 cup chopped parsley
- 1 pounds lamb, cubed

Instructions

Put ingredients in the slow cooker. Cover, and cook on low for 7 to 9 hours.

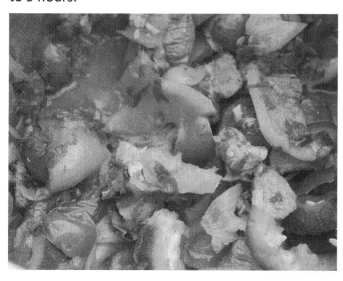

Plantain Chili

Serves 2

Ingredients - Allergies: SF, GF, DF, EF, NF

- 1 sliced plantain (1/2 inch thick sliced)
- 1/4 cup sliced carrot
- 1/2 cups chopped onions
- Salt, 1/4 Tsp. ground cayenne pepper and 1 Tsp. cumin seeds
- 2 Tbsp. corn
- 3/4 cup dry kidney beans
- 1/4 cup tomato paste
- 3/4 cup beef broth
- 1/4 tsp. ground coriander
- 1/4 cup chopped parsley
- 3/4 pound pork neck meat, cubed

Instructions

Put ingredients in the slow cooker. Cover, and cook on low for 7 to 9 hours.

BBQ Pork

Serves 2

Ingredients - Allergies: SF, GF, DF, EF, NF

- 1/2 cups tomato paste
- 1 Tbsp. lemon juice
- 2 tsp. mustard
- 1/4 tsp. ground black pepper
- 1/4 tsp. minced garlic
- Salt, 1 Tsp. ground cayenne pepper and 1 Tbsp. cumin seeds
- 1 pound pork neck meat

Instructions

Put ingredients in the slow cooker. Cover, and cook on low for 7 to 9 hours.

Penang Chicken Curry

Serves 2

Ingredients - Allergies: SF, GF, DF, EF, NF

- 1 pound chicken meat
- Curry Paste, but go low on the heat
- 1/4 cup tomato paste
- 1 Tsp. palm sugar (optional)
- 1 Tbsp. Thai basil leaves
- 1/4 cup coconut milk
- Cilantro or parsley for garnishing

Instructions

Put ingredients in the slow cooker. Cover, and cook on low for 7 to 9 hours.

Chicken Fennel Stew

Serves 2

Ingredients - Allergies: SF, GF, DF, EF, NF

- 1/2 cup sliced fennel (bulb and tops)
- 1/4 cup sliced carrot
- 1/2 cups chopped onions
- Salt, 1 Tsp. ground pepper and 1 minced garlic clove
- 1/2 cups chicken broth
- 1 Tbsp. chopped parsley
- 1 pound dark chicken meat

Instructions

Put ingredients in the slow cooker. Cover, and cook on low for 7 to 9 hours.

Garbanzo Kale Curry

Serves 2

Ingredients - Allergies: SF, GF, DF, EF, NF

- 1 cup dry garbanzo beans
- Curry Paste, but go low on the heat
- 1/4 cup sliced tomato
- 1 cup kale leaves
- 1/4 cup coconut milk

Instructions

Put ingredients in the slow cooker. Cover, and cook on low for 7 to 9 hours.

Mexican Veal

Serves 2

Ingredients - Allergies: SF, GF, DF, EF, NF

- 1/2 cups sliced carrot
- 1/2 cups chopped onions
- Salt, 1 Tsp. ground chili powder and 2 Tbsp. cumin seeds
- 1 Tbsp. tomato paste
- 1/2 cups beef broth
- 1 minced garlic clove
- 1 tsp. chili sauce
- 1 Tbsp. chopped mild green chiles
- 1 pound veal, cubed

Instructions

Put ingredients in the slow cooker. Cover, and cook on low for 7 to 9 hours.

Okra Pork Spinach Stew

Serves 2

Ingredients - Allergies: SF, GF, DF, EF, NF

- 1 cup okra
- 1/4 cup sliced carrot
- 1/2 cup chopped onions
- Salt, 1 Tsp. ground pepper
- 1/4 cup sliced tomatoes
- 1 cup spinach
- 1/4 cup tomato paste
- 1/2 cups beef broth
- 1 Tbsp. chopped parsley
- 1/2 pound pork neck meat, cubed

Instructions

Put ingredients in the slow cooker. Cover, and cook on low for 7 to 9 hours.

Red Curry

Serves 2

Ingredients - Allergies: SF, GF, DF, EF, NF

- 1 pound chicken meat
- Curry Paste, but go low on the heat
- 1/4 cup tomato paste
- 1 Tsp. palm sugar (optional)
- 1 Tsp. Thai basil leaves
- 1/4 cup sliced tomato
- 1/4 cup coconut milk
- Cilantro or parsley for garnishing

Instructions

Put ingredients in the slow cooker. Cover, and cook on low for 7 to 9 hours.

Shrimp & Green Peas

Serves 2

Ingredients - Allergies: SF, GF, DF, EF, NF

- 1/2 cup green peas
- 1/4 cup sliced carrot
- 1/2 cup chopped onions
- Salt & 1 Tsp. ground pepper to taste
- 1/4 cup tomato paste
- 1/4 cup fish broth
- 1 pound shrimp

Instructions

Put ingredients in the slow cooker. Cover, and cook on low for 5 to 6 hours.

Shrimp & Peppers

Serves 2

Ingredients - Allergies: SF, GF, DF, EF, NF

- 1/2 cup sliced red peppers
- 1/4 cup sliced carrot
- 1/2 cup chopped onions
- Salt & 1 Tsp. ground pepper to taste
- 1/2 cup sliced green peppers
- 1/4 cup tomato paste
- 1/2 cup fish broth
- 1 pound shrimp

Instructions

Put ingredients in the slow cooker. Cover, and cook on low for 5 to 6 hours.

BBQ Pork Ribs

Serves 2

Ingredients - Allergies: SF, GF, DF, EF, NF

- 1/2 cups tomato paste
- 1 Tbsp. lemon juice
- 1 tsp. mustard
- 1/8 tsp. salt
- 1/4 tsp. ground black pepper
- 1/4 tsp. minced garlic
- Salt, 1/4 Tsp. ground cayenne pepper and 1 Tsp. cumin seeds
- 1 pound pork ribs

Instructions

Put ingredients in the slow cooker. Cover, and cook on low for 7 to 9 hours. Serve with coleslaw.

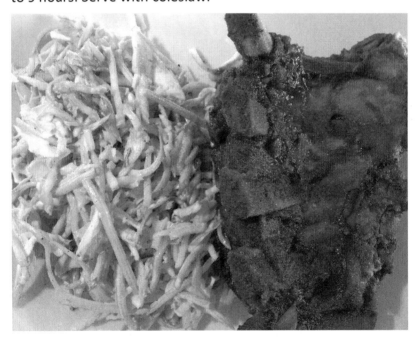

Pork Shoulder Stew

Serves 2

Ingredients - Allergies: SF, GF, DF, EF, NF

- 1/4 cup sliced red peppers
- 1/4 cup sliced carrot
- 1/2 cup sliced leeks
- Salt & 1 Tsp. ground pepper to taste
- 1 Tsp. cumin seeds & 1 bay leaf
- 1 garlic clove, minced
- 1 cup beef broth
- 1 pound pork shoulder

Instructions

Put ingredients in the slow cooker. Cover, and cook on low for 7 to 9 hours.

Fish, Onion & Fennel Stew

Serves 2

Ingredients - Allergies: SF, GF, DF, EF, NF

- 1/4 cup sliced yellow peppers
- 1/4 cup sliced carrot
- 1/2 cup chopped onions
- Salt & 1 Tsp. ground pepper to taste
- 1/2 cup sliced fennel bulb
- 1/4 cup tomato paste
- 1/4 cup fish broth
- 1 pound local fish

Instructions

Put ingredients in the slow cooker. Cover, and cook on low for 6 hours.

Kale & Shiitake Stew

Serves 2

Ingredients - Allergies: SF, GF, DF, EF, NF

- 1 garlic clove, minced
- 1/2 cups chopped onions
- 2 Tbsp. olive oil
- Salt & 1/4 Tsp. ground pepper to taste
- 1 cup vegetable broth
- 1/2 pound dry shiitake mushrooms

Instructions

Put ingredients in the slow cooker. Cover, and cook on low for 3 to 4 hours.

Kale & Chicken Stew

Serves 2

Ingredients - Allergies: SF, GF, DF, EF, NF

- 1/4 cup sliced leeks
- 1 sliced carrot
- 1/4 cup chopped onions
- Salt & 1/4 Tsp. ground pepper to taste
- 1/2 cups chicken broth
- 1 cup kale
- 1 pound chicken

Instructions

Put ingredients in the slow cooker. Cover, and cook on low for 7 to 9 hours.

Mackerel & Bamboo Shoots Stew

Serves 2

Ingredients - Allergies: SF, GF, DF, EF, NF

- 1/2 cup sliced bamboo shoots
- 1/2 cup sliced carrot
- 1/4 cup chopped onions
- Salt & 1 Tsp. ground pepper to taste
- 1/4 cup tomato paste
- 3/4 cup fish broth
- 1/4 cup chopped green onions for sprinkling
- 1 pound mackerel

Instructions

Put ingredients in the slow cooker. Cover, and cook on low for 5 to 6 hours.

Korean Spicy Fish Soup – Mae Un Tang

Serves 2

Ingredients - Allergies: SF, GF, DF, EF, NF

- 1/2 cup sliced daikon (radish)
- 13 garlic clove, minced
- 1/4 cup sliced green onions
- Salt & 1/4 Tsp. ground pepper to taste
- 1 Tsp. chopped ginger
- 2 Tsp. red pepper flakes (to taste)
- 1/4 cup tomato paste
- 1 + 1/2 cups water
- 1 pound local fish (pieces)

Instructions

Put ingredients in the slow cooker. Cover, and cook on low for 5 to 6 hours.

Mushrooms & Pork Ribs Stew

Serves 2

Ingredients - Allergies: SF, GF, DF, EF, NF

- 1 cup sliced bok choy
- 1/2 cup sliced mushrooms
- 1/2 cup chopped onions
- Salt & 1/5 Tsp. ground pepper to taste
- 1/2 cup beef broth
- 1 pound pork ribs

Instructions

Put ingredients in the slow cooker. Cover, and cook on low for 7 to 9 hours.

Olives Jambalaya

Serves 2

Ingredients - Allergies: SF, GF, DF, EF, NF

- 1/4 cup chopped onions & 1 minced garlic clove
- 1/2 tbsp. coconut oil & 1/4 tsp. turmeric
- Salt, ground black pepper to taste
- 3/4 pounds cubed chicken & 1/4 pound shrimp
- 1/4 tsp. dried red pepper flakes (to taste).
- 1 cup kale & 1/2 cup mushrooms
- 1/4 cup tomato paste & 1/4 cup chicken broth
- 1/2 cups Kalamata olives & 1 chopped carrot

Instructions

Put ingredients in the slow cooker. Cover, and cook on low for 7 to 9 hours.

Pork & Cauliflower Stew

Serves 2

Ingredients - Allergies: SF, GF, DF, EF, NF

- 1 cup sliced cauliflower
- 1 sliced carrot
- 1/2 cup chopped onions
- Salt & 1/4 Tsp. ground pepper to taste
- 1/2 cup beef broth
- 1 pound pork shoulder

Instructions

Put ingredients in the slow cooker. Cover, and cook on low for 7 to 9 hours.

Shui Zhu Yu - Sichuan Fish Stew

Serves 2

Ingredients - Allergies: SF, GF, DF, EF, NF

- 1/2 cup dried shiitake
- 1 Tsp. coconut oil
- 1/4 cup Chinese celery
- 1/4 Tsp. ground white pepper
- 3-5 dried chili red peppers (or more, to taste)
- Fish sauce or salt to taste & 1/4 Tsp. Sichuan peppercorns
- 1/4 cup sliced green onions
- 1 Tsp. minced ginger & 2 garlic cloves, minced
- 1 + 1/2 cups water
- 1 pounds local fish

Instructions

Put ingredients in the slow cooker. Cover, and cook on low for 5 to 6 hours.

Haleem – Beef & Lentils Stew

Serves 2

Ingredients - Allergies: SF, GF, DF, EF, NF

- 1 cup dry brown lentils
- 1/2 cup chopped onions & 1 garlic clove, minced
- Salt & 1 Tsp. ground pepper to taste
- 1 cup water
- 1 Tbsp. green chillies (to taste) & 1 Tsp. minced ginger
- 1/8 tsp. fenugreek seed, coriander, turmeric & cumin each
- 1/2 pound cubed beef (or mutton)
- 1 Tsp. cilantro leaves

Instructions

Put all ingredients except cilantro in the slow cooker. Cover, and cook on low for 7 to 9 hours. Sprinkle with cilantro and serve.

Hong Shao Rou Pork Stew

Serves 2

Ingredients - Allergies: SF, GF, DF, EF, NF

- 1 cup sliced leeks
- 1 sliced carrot
- 1 chopped green onion
- 1 Tsp. minced ginger
- Salt & 1/4 Tsp. ground pepper to taste
- 1/4 cup beef broth
- 1/2 cup red cooking wine
- 2 Tsp. fish sauce
- 1 pound pork belly, cubed

Instructions

Put all ingredients except green onions in the slow cooker. Cover, and cook on low for 7 to 9 hours. Sprinkle with green onions.

Pork Jambalaya

Serves 2

Ingredients - Allergies: SF, GF, DF, EF, NF

- 1/2 cups diced celery
- 1 sliced carrot
- 1/2 cup chopped onions & 1 clove minced garlic
- 1/2 cup sliced mushrooms
- Salt & 1/4 Tsp. ground pepper to taste
- 1/2 cups beef broth & 1/4 cup tomato paste
- 1/4 Tsp. red pepper flakes &
- 1 pound pork shoulder

Instructions

Put ingredients in the slow cooker. Cover, and cook on low for 7 to 9 hours.

Khoresht – Green Peas Stew

Serves 2

Ingredients - Allergies: SF, GF, DF, EF, NF

- 1/2 cups green peas
- 1 very small sliced eggplant
- 1/4 tsp. turmeric, cumin, cardamom each
- 1/2 cups chopped onions
- Salt & 1/4 Tsp. ground pepper to taste
- 1/4 cup chicken broth & 1/4 cup tomato paste
- 3/4 pound chicken breast meat

Instructions

Put ingredients in the slow cooker. Cover, and cook on low for 7 to 9 hours.

Kimchee Jjiagae – Kimchee Stew

Serves 2

Ingredients - Allergies: SF, GF, DF, EF, NF

- 1 cup kimchee
- 1/4 cup green peas
- 1 sliced green onion
- 1/4 cup chopped onions
- 1 Tsp. dried kelp
- 1/4 cup sliced radish
- Salt & 1/4 Tsp. ground pepper to taste
- 1/4 cup beef broth & 1/4 cup Tomato paste
- 1/4 tsp. red pepper flakes (to taste)
- 3/4 pound pork shoulder

Instructions

Put ingredients in the slow cooker. Cover, and cook on low for 7 to 9 hours.

Locro Argentine Stew

Serves 2

Ingredients - Allergies: SF, GF, DF, EF, NF

- 1/4 cup dry, broken hominy
- 1/2 cup dry white beans
- 1 cup sliced red peppers
- 1/2 cup chopped onions & 1 garlic clove, minced
- Salt & 1 Tsp. ground pepper to taste
- 3/4 cups beef broth
- 1/4 Tsp. cumin
- 1/2 pound Osso buco, cubed

Instructions

Put ingredients in the slow cooker. Cover, and cook on low for 7 to 9 hours.

Mixed Fish Stew

Serves 2

Ingredients - Allergies: SF, GF, DF, EF, NF

- 1/2 cups sliced red peppers
- 1/4 cup sliced celery
- 1/4 cup shredded carrot
- 1/4 cup white wine (optional)
- 1/2 cups chopped leeks
- Salt & 1 Tsp. ground pepper to taste
- 1 cup fish broth
- 1 pound fish steaks, mixed (e.g. salmon, cod etc.)

Instructions

Put ingredients in the slow cooker. Cover, and cook on low for 7 to 9 hours.

Onion, Leeks & Chicken Breast Stew

Serves 2

Ingredients - Allergies: SF, GF, DF, EF, NF

- 1/2 cups sliced leeks
- 1/4 cup shredded carrot
- 1/2 large onions, sliced in rings
- Salt & 1 Tsp. ground pepper to taste
- 3/4 cups chicken broth & 2 Tbsp. tomato paste
- 1 pound chicken breast meat

Instructions

Put ingredients in the slow cooker. Cover, and cook on low for 7 to 9 hours.

Pork & Onion Stew

Serves 2

Ingredients - Allergies: SF, GF, DF, EF, NF

- 1/2 cup sliced red onions
- 1/4 cup sliced carrot
- 1/2 cup chopped leeks
- Salt & 1 Tsp. ground pepper to taste
- 1/2 cup beef broth
- 1 pound pork shoulder

Instructions

Put ingredients in the slow cooker. Cover, and cook on low for 7 to 9 hours.

Shrimp Gumbo Stew

Serves 2

Ingredients - Allergies: SF, GF, DF, EF, NF

- 1/4 cup chopped celery
- 1/4 cup sliced red peppers
- 1/4 cup sliced carrot
- 1/2 cups chopped onions
- Salt & 1 Tsp. ground pepper to taste
- 1/2 cups fish broth & 1/4 cup tomato paste
- 1/4 pound cubed chicken
- 3/4 pounds shrimp

Instructions

Put ingredients in the slow cooker. Cover, and cook on low for 7 to 9 hours.

Cholent – Jewish Brisket & Beans Stew

Serves 2

Ingredients - Allergies: SF, GF, DF, EF, NF

- 1/2 cups diced celery
- 1/4 cup sliced carrot
- 1/2 cup chopped onions & 1 cloves minced garlic
- 1/4 cup dried butter beans
- 1/4 cup dried kidney beans
- Salt & 1 Tsp. ground pepper to taste
- 1 cups water or beef broth
- 1/4 Tsp. red pepper flakes (to taste)
- 3/4 pounds beef brisket, cubed

Instructions

Put ingredients in the slow cooker. Cover, and cook on low for 7 to 9 hours.

Beef Daube Stew

Serves 2

Ingredients - Allergies: SF, GF, DF, EF, NF

- 1/4 cup mushrooms & 1 small rosemary spring
- 1/4 cup sliced carrot & 1 thyme sprigs
- 1/2 cup chopped onions & 1 cloves minced garlic
- Salt & 1 Tsp. ground pepper to taste
- 1/4 cup beef broth & 1/4 cup tomato paste
- 1/4 Tsp. red pepper flakes
- 1 pound beef chuck, cubed

Instructions

Put ingredients in the slow cooker. Cover, and cook on low for 7 to 9 hours.

Dinuguan – Filipino Stew

Serves 2

Ingredients - Allergies: SF, GF, DF, EF, NF

- 1/4 cup sliced green peppers
- 1/4 cup sliced carrot
- 1/2 cup chopped onions & 1 clove minced garlic
- 2 Tbsp. vinegar
- Salt & 1 Tsp. ground pepper to taste
- 3/4 cups beef broth or water
- 1 Tsp. minced ginger
- 1/2 pounds pork shoulder, cubed
- 1/4 pound pork liver, cubed
- 1/4 pound pork kidney (optionally swap with liver or pork shoulder)

Instructions

Put ingredients in the slow cooker. Cover, and cook on low for 7 to 9 hours.

Fabada Asturiana – Spanish Pork Belly & Beans Stew

Serves 2

Ingredients - Allergies: SF, GF, DF, EF, NF

- 1/2 cup chopped onions & 1 cloves minced garlic
- 1/2 cup dried butter beans
- Salt & 1 Tsp. ground pepper to taste
- 1/2 cups beef broth
- 1/4 cup kale
- 1/4 Tsp. saffron
- 1 pound pork belly, cubed

Instructions

Put ingredients in the slow cooker. Cover, and cook on low for 7 to 9 hours.

Ghormeh Sabzi – Persian Stew

Serves 2

Ingredients - Allergies: SF, GF, DF, EF, NF

- 3/4 cup spinach or kale
- 1/4 cup sliced green onions
- 1/4 cup chopped onions & 1 clove minced garlic
- 1 tsp. minced ginger
- Salt & 1 Tsp. ground pepper to taste
- 1/2 cups beef broth
- 2 Tbsp. lemon juice
- 1/4 Tsp. turmeric
- 1/4 cup cilantro
- 1/4 cup parsley
- 1 pound lamb or beef stewing meat

Instructions

Put ingredients in the slow cooker. Cover, and cook on low for 7 to 9 hours.

Goulash – Spicy Beef Stew
Serves 2

Ingredients - Allergies: SF, GF, DF, EF, NF

- 1 cup diced celery
- 1 shredded carrot
- 1/2 cup chopped onions & 1 clove minced garlic
- 2 Tsp. sweet paprika
- Salt & 1/4 Tsp. ground pepper to taste
- 1 cup beef broth & 1/4 cup tomato paste
- 1/4 Tsp. red pepper flakes
- 1 pound beef stew meat
- 1 Tsp. chopped parsley

Instructions

Put ingredients in the slow cooker. Cover, and cook on low for 7 to 9 hours. Sprinkle with parsley.

Letscho Chicken

Serves 2

Ingredients - Allergies: SF, GF, DF, EF, NF

- 1/2 cup sliced green peppers
- 1/2 cup chopped onions & 1 clove minced garlic
- 1/2 cup sliced red peppers
- Salt & 1/4 Tsp. ground pepper to taste
- 1 tomato, sliced
- 1/4 Tsp. red pepper flakes
- 2 Tsp. sweet paprika
- 1/2 cup green beans
- 1 pound chicken meat, cubed

Instructions

Put ingredients in the slow cooker. Cover, and cook on low for 7 to 9 hours.

Narial Murgh Shorba Stew

Serves 2

Ingredients - Allergies: SF, GF, DF, EF, NF

- 1/2 cup diced celery
- 1/4 cup curry paste (see recipe at the beginning of the book)
- 1/2 cup chopped onions & 1 clove minced garlic
- 1/2 cup sliced mushrooms
- Salt & 1/4 Tsp. ground pepper to taste
- 1 cup water
- 1 pound chicken meat

Instructions

Put ingredients in the slow cooker. Cover, and cook on low for 7 to 9 hours.

Pibil Pollo – Mexican Chicken Stew

Serves 2

Ingredients - Allergies: SF, GF, DF, EF, NF

- 1/2 cups shredded celery
- 1 shredded carrot
- 1/2 cup chopped onions & 1 clove minced garlic
- 1/4 cup grapefruit juice
- Salt & 1/4 Tsp. ground pepper to taste
- 1/2 cup chicken broth & ½ small diced tomato
- 25 gr. of anchiote paste
- 1 pound chicken dark meat, boneless, skinless
- 1/4 tsp. ground cumin

Instructions

Put ingredients in the slow cooker. Cover, and cook on low for 7 to 9 hours.

Palak Daal - Spinach Lentil Stew

Serves 2

Ingredients - Allergies: SF, GF, DF, EF, NF

- 1 cup spinach or kale, chopped
- 1/4 cup curry paste
- 1 Tbsp. coconut oil
- 1/2 cup chopped onions & 1 clove minced garlic
- 1 cup dried lentils
- Salt & 1/4 Tsp. ground pepper to taste
- 1 cups water
- 1/4 Tsp. red pepper flakes
- 2 Tsp. lemon juice

Instructions

Put ingredients in the slow cooker. Cover, and cook on low for 7 to 9 hours.

Four Mushrooms Stew

Serves 2

Ingredients - Allergies: SF, GF, DF, EF, NF

- 3/4 cup sliced leeks
- 1/4 cup chopped onion
- Salt & 1/4 Tsp. ground pepper to taste
- 1 small tomato, sliced
- 1 Tbsp. parsley
- 1/4 cup vegetable broth
- 1/4 pound dry shiitake mushrooms
- 1/4 pound Portobello mushrooms, sliced
- 1/4 pound oyster mushrooms, sliced
- 1/4 pound cremini mushrooms, sliced
- 1 Tsp. Thyme and Sage each

Instructions

Put ingredients in the slow cooker. Cover, and cook on low for 5 to 6 hours.

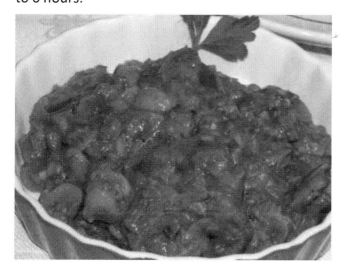

Birria Stew – Mexican (Jalisco) Beef Stew

Serves 2

Ingredients - Allergies: SF, GF, DF, EF, NF

- 1/2 cup chopped onion & 1 clove minced garlic
- 2 tomatoes, sliced
- Salt & 1/4 Tsp. ground pepper to taste
- 1/4 ancho and guajillo chilies each
- 1 Tsp. cumin
- 1 bay leaf
- 1/2 cup beef broth
- 1 pound beef meat, cubed or lamb (optionally)

Instructions

Put ingredients in the slow cooker. Cover, and cook on low for 7 to 9 hours.

Chanko Nabe Stew

Serves 2

Ingredients - Allergies: SF, GF, DF, EF, NF

- 1/4 cup Shimeji and enoki mushrooms each (or shiitake)
- 1 Tbsp. dried kombu seaweed
- Salt & 1/4 Tsp. ground pepper to taste
- 1/4 cup green onions, sliced & 1 Tbsp. minced onion
- 1/4 cup bok choy, sliced
- 1 carrot, sliced
- 1/4 cup napa cabbage, sliced
- 2 Tsp. fish sauce
- 1 Tsp. miso paste (optional)
- 1 Tsp. minced ginger
- 1 + ½ cup fish broth
- 1/2 pounds ground pork & 1 egg for meatballs
- 1/2 pound shrimp

Instructions

Make meatballs by mixing ground pork, 1 Tsp. fish sauce , 1 egg & 1 Tbsp. minced onion. Put ingredients in the slow cooker. Cover, and cook on low for 7 to 9 hours.

Fava Beans Stew

Serves 2

Ingredients - Allergies: SF, GF, DF, EF, NF

- •3/4 cup sliced red peppers and leaks, each
- 1/2 cup chopped onions & 1 clove minced garlic
- Salt & 1/4 Tsp. ground pepper to taste
- 1 tomato, sliced
- 1 Tsp. dried chilies & 1 Tsp. cumin
- 2 Tsp. sweet paprika
- 2 cups water
- 1/2 pound dried fava beans & 1/2 pound pork neck meat

Instructions

Put ingredients in the slow cooker. Cover, and cook on low for 7 to 9 hours.

Lamb, Basil, Parsley & Tomato Stew

Serves 2

Ingredients - Allergies: SF, GF, DF, EF, NF

- 1/2 cup chopped onions & 1 clove minced garlic
- 1/2 cup sliced red peppers
- Salt & 1/4 Tsp. ground pepper to taste
- 1 tomato, sliced or 3/4 cup cherry tomatoes
- 1 Tbsp. basil leaves
- 1/4 cup chopped parsley
- 1 pound lamb meat, cubed

Instructions

Put ingredients in the slow cooker. Cover, and cook on low for 7 to 9 hours.

Spicy Mexican Chicken Stew

Serves 2

Ingredients - Allergies: SF, GF, DF, EF, NF

- 3/4 cup sliced leeks
- 1/4 cup chopped onions & 1 clove minced garlic
- 1/2 cup sliced red peppers
- Salt & 1/4 Tsp. ground pepper to taste
- 1 tomato, sliced
- 1 Tsp. chipotle
- 1 Tsp. cumin
- 1 Tbsp. cup cilantro
- 1 pound chicken meat, cubed

Instructions

Put ingredients in the slow cooker. Cover, and cook on low for 7 to 9 hours.

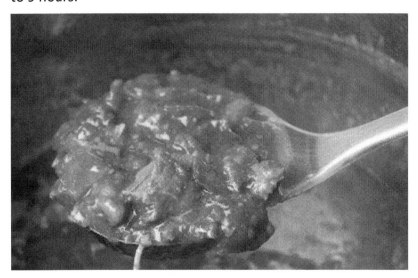

Szekely Stew

Serves 2

Ingredients - Allergies: SF, GF, DF, EF, NF

- 1 cup sliced sauerkraut
- 1/2 cup chopped onions & 1 clove minced garlic
- Salt & 1/4 Tsp. ground pepper to taste
- 1 Tsp. caraway seeds
- 1 Tsp. chopped parsley for decoration
- 1/4 Tsp. red pepper flakes
- 1 Tbsp. sweet paprika
- 1 pound pork shoulder meat, cubed

Instructions

Put ingredients in the slow cooker. Cover, and cook on low for 7 to 9 hours. Decorate with parsley.

Veal, Carrot & Cauliflower Stew

Serves 2

Ingredients - Allergies: SF, GF, DF, EF, NF

- 3/4 cup cauliflower florets
- 1/2 cup chopped onions & 1 clove minced garlic
- 1/2 cup sliced red peppers
- Salt & 1/4 Tsp. ground pepper to taste
- 1 carrot, sliced
- 1/2 Tsp. red pepper flakes
- 2 Tsp. sweet paprika
- 1 pound veal meat, cubed

Instructions

Put ingredients in the slow cooker. Cover, and cook on low for 7 to 9 hours.

Venison & Basil Stew

Serves 2

Ingredients - Allergies: SF, GF, DF, EF, NF

- 1/2 cup chopped onions & 1 clove minced garlic
- 1/2 cup sliced red peppers
- Salt & 1/4 Tsp. ground pepper to taste
- 1 tomato, sliced
- 1/4 Tsp. red pepper flakes
- 2 Tsp. sweet paprika
- 1/4 cup basil leaves
- 3/4 cups beef broth
- 1 pound venison meat, cubed

Instructions

Put ingredients in the slow cooker. Cover, and cook on low for 7 to 9 hours.

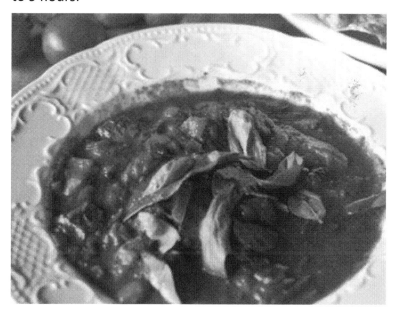

Venison & Cauliflower Stew

Serves 2

Ingredients - Allergies: SF, GF, DF, EF, NF

- 1/2 cup cauliflower florets
- 1/2 cup chopped onions & 1 clove minced garlic
- 1/2 cup sliced red peppers
- Salt & 1/4 Tsp. ground pepper to taste
- 1 tomato, sliced
- 1/4 Tsp. red pepper flakes
- 1 Tsp. sweet paprika
- 3/4 cup beef broth
- 1 pound chicken meat, cubed

Instructions

Put ingredients in the slow cooker. Cover, and cook on low for 7 to 9 hours.

Beef Eintopf - German Beef Stew

Serves 2

Ingredients - Allergies: SF, GF, DF, EF, NF

- 1/4 cup cauliflower florets
- 1/2 cup chopped onions & 1 clove minced garlic
- 1/4 cup sliced carrots
- Salt & 1/4 Tsp. ground pepper to taste
- 1/4 cup green beans
- 1/4 cup green peas
- 3/4 cup beef broth
- 1 pounds beef stew meat, cubed

Instructions

Put ingredients in the slow cooker. Cover, and cook on low for 7 to 9 hours.

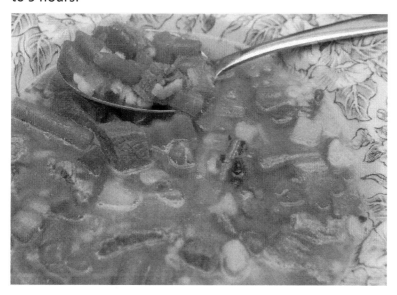

Bo Kho – Vietnamese Beef Stew

Serves 2

Ingredients - Allergies: SF, GF, DF, EF, NF

- 1/2 cup sliced carrots
- 1/2 cup chopped onions & 1 Tsp. minced ginger
- 3/4 cup sliced tomatoes & 1 small bay leaf
- Salt & 1/4 Tsp. ground pepper to taste
- 1 teaspoon curry paste
- 1/4 Tsp. red pepper flakes
- 1 Tbsp. fish sauce & 1 small star anise, whole
- 3/4 cup beef broth & 1/4 stalk lemongrass
- 1 pound beef brisket, cubed

Instructions

Put ingredients in the slow cooker. Cover, and cook on low for 7 to 9 hours.

Brunswick Stew

Serves 2

Ingredients - Allergies: SF, GF, DF, EF, NF

- 1/4 cup dry butterbeans
- 1/2 cup chopped onion & 1 clove minced garlic
- 1/2 cup okra
- Salt & 1/4 Tsp. ground pepper to taste
- 1 tomato, sliced
- 1/4 cup sliced celery and carrots each
- 2 Tsp. sweet paprika
- 3/4 cup beef broth
- 1 pound chicken or pork meat, cubed

Instructions

Put ingredients in the slow cooker. Cover, and cook on low for 7 to 9 hours.

Caldeirada De Peixe - Portuguese Fish Stew

Serves 2

Ingredients - Allergies: SF, GF, DF, EF, NF

- 1/4 cup green peas
- 1/2 cup chopped onions & 1 clove minced garlic
- 1/4 cup sliced red peppers and carrots each
- Salt & 1/4 Tsp. ground pepper to taste
- 1 tomato, sliced
- 1 Tsp. cilantro, for sprinkling
- 1/4-pound shrimp and mussels, each
- 3/4 cups fish broth
- 1/4 pound swordfish and haddock, each

Instructions

Put ingredients in the slow cooker. Cover, and cook on low for 7 to 9 hours. Sprinkle with cilantro.

Cassoulet – French Pork & Bean Stew

Serves 2

Ingredients - Allergies: SF, GF, DF, EF, NF

- 1/2 cup dry cannellini beans
- 1/2 cup chopped onions & 1 clove minced garlic
- 1/4 cup sliced carrot
- Salt & 1/4 Tsp. ground pepper to taste
- 1/4 cup celery, sliced
- 1 Tsp. parsley
- 1 Tsp. sweet paprika
- 1 cup chicken broth
- 1/2 pounds cubed pork meat and chicken drumsticks, each

Instructions

Put ingredients in the slow cooker. Cover, and cook on low for 7 to 9 hours.

Chicken & Lentil Stew

Serves 2

Ingredients - Allergies: SF, GF, DF, EF, NF

- 1 cup sliced carrots
- 2 cups chopped onions & 2 cloves minced garlic
- 2 cup dry lentils
- Salt & 1 Tsp. ground pepper to taste
- 1 cup red peppers
- 1 cup green peas
- 2 Tbsp. sweet paprika
- 2 cups chicken broth
- 4 pounds chicken meat, cubed

Instructions

Put ingredients in the slow cooker. Cover, and cook on low for 7 to 9 hours.

Chorba – Beef or Lamb Stew

Serves 2

Ingredients - Allergies: SF, GF, DF, EF, NF

- 1/2 cup sliced celery & 1 Tsp. minced ginger
- 1/2 cup chopped onions & 1 clove minced garlic
- 1/4 cup parsley and cilantro each
- Salt & 1 Tsp. ground pepper to taste
- 1 tomato, sliced
- 1/4 Tsp. red pepper flakes and turmeric each
- 1 sliced carrot
- 1 cup beef broth
- 1 pound beef or lamb meat, cubed
- 1/4 cup dry chickpeas

Instructions

Put ingredients in the slow cooker. Cover, and cook on low for 7 to 9 hours.

Eintopf – Lentil, Carrot, Beans & Peppers Stew

Serves 2

Ingredients - Allergies: SF, GF, DF, EF, NF

- 1 sliced carrot
- 1/2 cup chopped onions & 1 clove minced garlic
- 1/2 cup sliced red peppers
- Salt & 1 Tsp. ground pepper to taste
- 1 tomato, sliced
- 1/4 Tsp. red pepper flakes
- 1/2 cup lentils
- 3/4 cup beef broth
- 1/2 pounds pork meat, cubed

Instructions

Put ingredients in the slow cooker. Cover, and cook on low for 7 to 9 hours.

Ewedu -Nigerian Mallow Leaves Stew

Serves 2

Ingredients - Allergies: SF, GF, DF, EF, NF

- 1 cup mallow leaves – optionally 1/2 cup grape leaves, 1/2 cup kale or spinach – blended if you want
- 1/2 cup chopped onions & 1 clove minced garlic
- 1/2 cup sliced mushrooms
- Salt & 1 Tsp. ground pepper to taste
- 1/4 Tsp. red pepper flakes
- 1/2 cup fish broth
- 1 pound shrimp

Instructions

This Is modified original Ewedu recipe. Put ingredients in the slow cooker. Cover, and cook on low for 7 to 9 hours.

Lamb Liver Stew

Serves 2

Ingredients - Allergies: SF, GF, DF, EF, NF

- 1 cup cauliflower florets
- 1/2 cup chopped onions & 1 clove minced garlic
- 1/2 cup sliced red peppers
- Salt & 1 Tsp. ground pepper to taste
- 1 tomato, sliced
- 1/4 Tsp. red pepper flakes
- 2 Tsp. sweet paprika
- 1 cups beef broth
- 1 pounds lamb liver, cubed

Instructions

Put ingredients in the slow cooker. Cover, and cook on low for 7 to 9 hours.

Pork Neck Chili

Serves 2

Ingredients - Allergies: SF, GF, DF, EF, NF

- 2 tsp. coconut oil
- 1 onion, chopped
- 1 clove garlic, minced
- 1/4 pound ground pork
- 1/4-pound pork neck meat, cubed
- 1 diced tomato
- 1/4 cup strong brewed coffee
- 1/4 cup tomato paste
- 3/4 cups beef broth
- 1 tsp. cumin seeds
- 1/2 tsp. dried oregano
- 1/2 tsp. ground cayenne pepper
- 1/2 tsp. ground coriander
- 1/2 tsp. salt
- 1/2 cup dry kidney beans
- 1/2 cup dry navy beans
- 1 fresh hot chili pepper, chopped

Instructions

Put ingredients in the slow cooker. Cover, and cook on low for 7 to 9 hours.

Lentil Kale Stew

Serves 2

Ingredients - Allergies: SF, GF, DF, EF, NF

- 1/2 cup chopped onions
- 2 tsp. coconut oil
- 1 cup chopped Kale
- 1 tomato
- Salt, ground black pepper and ground cumin to taste
- 1 cup beef stock
- 1 cups dry lentils

Instructions

Put ingredients in the slow cooker. Cover, and cook on low for 7 to 9 hours.

Lentil & Leeks Stew

Serves 2

Ingredients - Allergies: SF, GF, DF, EF, NF

- 1 cup chopped leeks
- 2 tsp. coconut oil
- 1 carrot, chopped
- 3/4 cup celery, chopped
- Salt, ground black pepper and ground cumin to taste
- 1 cup vegetable stock
- 1 Tbsp. chopped parsley
- 1 cup dry lentils

Instructions

Put ingredients in the slow cooker. Cover, and cook on low for 7 to 9 hours.

Octopus Stew

Serves 2

Ingredients - Allergies: SF, GF, DF, EF, NF

- 1/2 cups chopped onions & 2 garlic cloves, minced
- 2 tbsp. coconut oil
- 1 red tomato, chopped
- 1/2 red pepper, chopped
- 1 carrot, chopped & 1 bay leaf
- 3 olives & 1 Tbsp. lemon juice
- Salt, ground black pepper to taste
- 1/2 cups fish stock
- 1 Tbsp. chopped parsley & dill, each
- 1 pound octopus or baby octopus pieces

Instructions

Put ingredients in the slow cooker. Cover, and cook on low for 7 to 9 hours.

Pork, Green Peppers & Tomato Stew

Serves 2

Ingredients - Allergies: SF, GF, DF, EF, NF

- 1/2 cup chopped onions
- 1 tbsp. coconut oil
- 1 tomato, chopped
- 1 green pepper, chopped
- Salt, ground black pepper to taste
- 1/4 cup beef stock
- 1 pound pork meat, cubed

Instructions

Put ingredients in the slow cooker. Cover, and cook on low for 7 to 9 hours.

Pork Neck and Peppers Stew

Serves 2

Ingredients - Allergies: SF, GF, DF, EF, NF

- 1/2 cup chopped onions
- 1 tbsp. coconut oil
- 2 carrots, chopped
- 1 green pepper, chopped
- Salt, ground black pepper and ground cumin to taste
- 1 cups beef stock
- 1 Tbsp. cup chopped parsley & 1 bay leaf
- 1/2 cup chopped celery
- 1 pound pork neck meat, cubed

Instructions

Put ingredients in the slow cooker. Cover, and cook on low for 7 to 9 hours.

Pork, Peppers & Green Peas Stew

Serves 2

Ingredients - Allergies: SF, GF, DF, EF, NF

- 1/2 cup chopped onions
- 1 tbsp. coconut oil
- 1 tomato, chopped
- 1 red pepper, chopped
- 1/4 cup green peas
- Salt, ground black pepper and ground cumin to taste
- 1/2 cups beef stock
- 1/2 cup sliced celery
- 1 pound pork, cubed

Instructions

Put ingredients in the slow cooker. Cover, and cook on low for 7 to 9 hours.

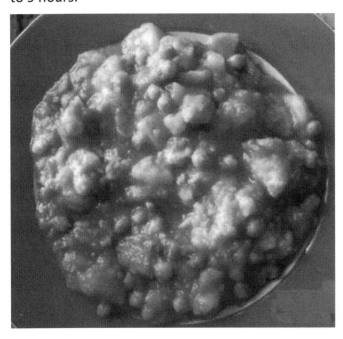

Veal and Peppers Stew

Serves 2

Ingredients - Allergies: SF, GF, DF, EF, NF

- 1/2 cup chopped onions
- 1 tbsp. coconut oil
- 1 red pepper, chopped
- 1 tomato, chopped
- Salt, ground black pepper and ground cumin to taste
- 1 cup beef stock
- 1/2 cauliflower
- 1 pound veal, cubed

Instructions

Put ingredients in the slow cooker. Cover, and cook on low for 7 to 9 hours.

Venison and Carrots Stew

Serves 2

Ingredients - Allergies: SF, GF, DF, EF, NF

- 1/2 cup chopped onions
- 1 tbsp. coconut oil
- 1 small red pepper, chopped
- 1 tomato, chopped
- Salt, ground black pepper and ground cumin to taste
- 3/4 cups beef stock
- 1/2 cup cauliflower
- 1 pound venison, cubed

Instructions

Put ingredients in the slow cooker. Cover, and cook on low for 7 to 9 hours.

Pork & Sweet Potato Stew

Serves 2

Ingredients - Allergies: SF, GF, DF, EF, NF

- 1/2 cup chopped onions
- 1 tbsp. coconut oil
- 1 small red pepper, chopped
- 1 cup celery, chopped
- 1/2 cup sweet potato, chopped
- Salt, ground black pepper and ground cumin to taste
- 3/4 cup beef stock
- 1 cup cauliflower
- 1 pound lamb, cubed

Instructions

Put ingredients in the slow cooker. Cover, and cook on low for 7 to 9 hours.

Beef, Carrots & Eggplant Stew

Serves 2

Ingredients - Allergies: SF, GF, DF, EF, NF

- 1/2 cup chopped onions & 1 minced garlic clove
- 1 tbsp. coconut oil & 2 bay leaves
- Salt, ground black pepper and ground cumin to taste
- 1 pound cubed beef stew meat
- 1 quartered carrot
- 3/4 cup sliced eggplant
- 1/2 cup beef broth

Instructions

Put ingredients in the slow cooker. Cover, and cook on low for 8 hours.

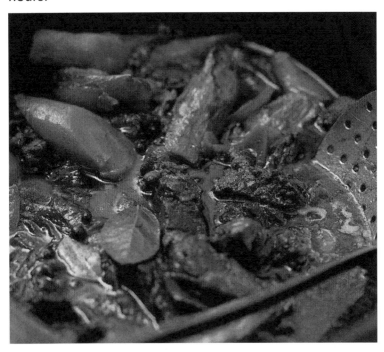

Beef, Cauliflower & Carrots Stew

Serves 2

Ingredients - Allergies: SF, GF, DF, EF, NF

- 1/2 cup chopped onions & 1 minced garlic clove
- 1 tbsp. coconut oil
- Salt, ground black pepper to taste
- 1 pound cubed beef stew meat
- 3/4 cup cauliflower florets
- 1/2 cup sliced celery
- 1 sliced carrot
- 1 Tbsp. sliced parsley
- 1 Tbsp. paprika
- 1/2 cup beef broth

Instructions

Put ingredients in the slow cooker. Cover, and cook on low for 8 hours.

Pork Meat & Liver Stew

Serves 2

Ingredients - Allergies: SF, GF, DF, EF, NF

- 1 sliced red pepper
- 1 sliced carrot
- 1/2 cup chopped onions & 1 minced garlic clove
- 1 Tbsp. vinegar
- Salt & 1 Tsp. ground pepper to taste
- 3/4 cups beef broth or water
- 1 Tsp. minced ginger
- 1/2 pound pork shoulder, cubed
- 1/4 pound pork liver, cubed
- 1/4 pound pork kidney (or pork liver or pork shoulder)

Instructions

Put ingredients in the slow cooker. Cover, and cook on low for 8 hours.

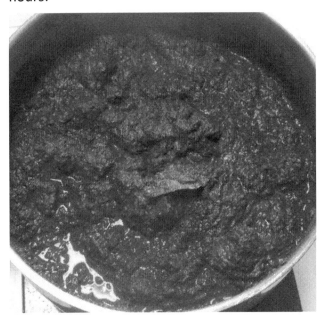

Gumbo Chicken

Serves 2

Ingredients - Allergies: SF, GF, DF, EF, NF

- 1/2 cup chopped celery
- 1 sliced red peppers
- 1 sliced carrot
- 1/2 cup chopped onions
- Salt & 1 Tsp. ground pepper to taste
- 3/4 cups chicken broth & 1 Tbsp. tomato paste
- 3/4 pound cubed chicken
- 1/4 pound shrimp

Instructions

Put ingredients in the slow cooker. Cover, and cook on low for 8 hours.

Sauerkraut Pork Stew

Serves 2

Ingredients - Allergies: SF, GF, DF, EF, NF

- 1 cup sauerkraut
- 1 Tbsp. cup green peas
- 1/2 cup chopped onions
- 1 Tbsp. cup sliced radish
- Salt & 1 Tsp. ground pepper to taste
- 1/4 cup beef broth & 2 Tsp. paprika
- 1 tsp. red pepper flakes (to taste)
- 1 pound pork shoulder

Instructions

Put ingredients in the slow cooker. Cover, and cook on low for 8 hours.

Lamb, Carrots & Cauliflower Stew

Serves 2

Ingredients - Allergies: SF, GF, DF, EF, NF

- 1/2 cup chopped onions
- 1 tbsp. coconut oil
- Salt, ground black pepper to taste
- 1 pound cubed lamb
- 1/4 cup sliced celery
- 1/2 cup cauliflower florets
- 1 sliced carrot
- 1 Tbsp. paprika
- 1/2 cup beef broth

Instructions

Put ingredients in the slow cooker. Cover, and cook on low for 8 hours.

Mixed Seafood Stew

Serves 2

Ingredients - Allergies: SF, GF, DF, EF, NF

- 1/2 cups chopped onions
- 2 tbsp. coconut oil
- 1 sliced tomato
- Salt, 2 Tbsp. chopped dill.
- 1 cup fish or vegetable stock
- 1/4 pound shrimp
- 1/4 pound mussels
- 1/2 pounds local fish

Instructions

Put ingredients in the slow cooker. Cover, and cook on low for 8 hours.

Navy Beans Stew

Serves 2

Ingredients - Allergies: SF, GF, DF, EF, NF

- 1/2 cups diced celery
- 2 sliced carrots
- 1 chopped onion & 1 clove minced garlic
- 1/2 cups dry navy beans & 1/4 tsp. cumin
- Salt & 1 Tsp. ground pepper to taste
- 1 cup water or beef broth
- 1/4 Tsp. red pepper flakes (to taste)
- 1/4 pound beef brisket, cubed
- 1/4 pound pork neck meat, cubed

Instructions

Put ingredients in the slow cooker. Cover, and cook on low for 8 hours.

Veal, Cauliflower & Mushrooms Stew

Serves 2

Ingredients - Allergies: SF, GF, DF, EF, NF

- 1 chopped onion & 1 minced garlic clove
- 2 tbsp. coconut oil
- Salt, ground black pepper to taste
- 1 pound veal
- 1/2 cup Portobello mushrooms
- 1/2 cup cauliflower florets
- 1/2 cup beef broth
- 1 Tbsp. parsley

Instructions

Put ingredients in the slow cooker. Cover, and cook on low for 8 hours.

Veal, Carrots & Mushrooms Stew

Serves 2

Ingredients - Allergies: SF, GF, DF, EF, NF

- 1 chopped onion & 1 minced garlic clove
- 2 tbsp. coconut oil
- Salt, ground black pepper to taste
- 1 pound veal
- 1/2 cups Portobello mushrooms
- 1 carrot
- 1/2 cups beef broth
- 1 Tbsp. parsley

Instructions

Put ingredients in the slow cooker. Cover, and cook on low for 8 hours.

Hunters stew

Serves 2

Ingredients - Allergies: SF, GF, DF, EF, NF

- 1 chopped onion
- 2 tbsp. coconut oil
- Salt, ground black pepper to taste
- 1/2 pound pork shoulder meat, cubed
- 1/2 pound venison meat, cubed
- 1/2 cup shredded cabbage
- 1/2 cups sauerkraut cabbage
- 1 minced garlic clove
- 1 Tsp. ground paprika

Instructions

Put ingredients in the slow cooker. Cover, and cook on low for 9 hours.

Laos beef and tripe stew

Serves 2

Ingredients - Allergies: SF, GF, DF, EF, NF

- 2 sliced carrots
- 2 chopped onions & 1 Tbsp. minced ginger
- 2 sliced tomatoes & 1/2 bay leaf
- Salt & 1 Tsp. ground pepper to taste
- 1 teaspoon curry paste
- 1/4 Tsp. red pepper flakes
- 1 Tbsp. fish sauce & 1 star anise, whole
- 1/2 cups beef broth & 1/4 stalk lemongrass
- 1/2 pounds beef brisket and beef tripe each

Instructions

Put ingredients in the slow cooker. Cover, and cook on low for 9 hours.

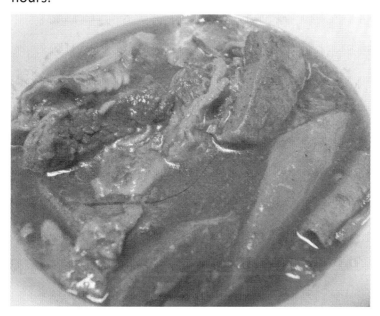

Chili Con Carne

Serves 2

Ingredients - Allergies: SF, GF, DF, EF, NF

- 2 tbsp. coconut oil
- 1 onion, chopped
- 1 clove garlic, minced
- 3/4 pounds minced beef meat
- 1 Tbsp. corn, chopped green and red pepper each
- 1 tomato
- 3/4 cups beef broth
- 1 tsp. cumin seeds
- 1/4 tsp. ground cayenne pepper
- 1/4 tsp. ground coriander
- 1/4 tsp. salt
- 3/4 cups dry kidney beans
- 1 fresh hot chili pepper, chopped

Instructions

Put ingredients in the slow cooker. Cover, and cook on low for 9 hours.

Lentil & Leafy Veggies Stew

Serves 2

Ingredients - Allergies: SF, GF, DF, EF, NF

- 1/4 cup chopped kale, leeks and Swiss Chard each
- 2 tbsp. coconut oil
- 1 carrot, chopped
- 1 cup celery, chopped
- Salt, ground black pepper and ground cumin to taste
- 1 cup vegetable stock
- 1 Tbsp. chopped parsley
- 1 cup dry lentils

Instructions

Put ingredients in the slow cooker. Cover, and cook on low for 9 hours.

Mushrooms & Lamb stew

Serves 2

Ingredients - Allergies: SF, GF, DF, EF, NF

- 1 cup sliced Portobello mushrooms
- 1/4 cup green beans
- 2 chopped onions
- 2 tbsp. coconut oil
- Salt, ground black pepper and ground cumin to taste
- 1 bay leaf & 1 Tsp. chopped garlic
- 1/2 cup beef stock & 1 Tbsp. tomato paste
- 1 pound lamb, cubed

Instructions

Put ingredients in the slow cooker. Cover, and cook on low for 9 hours.

Pork and Green Peppers stew

Serves 2

Ingredients - Allergies: SF, GF, DF, EF, NF

- 1/2 cups green peppers, sliced
- 1/4 cup red peppers, sliced
- 2 chopped onions
- 2 tbsp. coconut oil
- Salt, ground black pepper and ground cumin to taste
- 1 bay leaf & 1 Tsp. chopped garlic
- 1/2 cups beef stock & 1 Tsp. paprika
- 1 pound pork shoulder

Instructions

Put ingredients in the slow cooker. Cover, and cook on low for 9 hours.

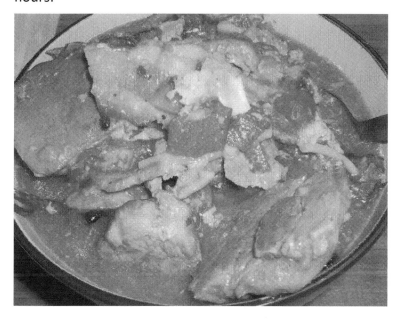

Spezzatino di Vitello – Italian veal stew
Serves 2

Ingredients - Allergies: SF, GF, DF, EF, NF

- 1 carrot
- 1 tomato, quartered
- 2 chopped onions
- 2 tbsp. coconut oil
- Salt, ground black pepper and ground cumin to taste
- 1 mint leaf & 2 Tsp. chopped garlic
- 1/2 cups beef stock
- 1 pound veal

Instructions

Put ingredients in the slow cooker. Cover, and cook on low for 9 hours.

Tomato Fish stew

Serves 2

Ingredients - Allergies: SF, GF, DF, EF, NF

- 1 sliced tomato
- 1 small shredded carrot
- 2 chopped onions
- Salt & 1 Tsp. ground pepper to taste
- 1/4 cup chopped parsley (save 1 tsp. for decoration)
- 1/2 cup fish broth
- 1 pound mixed local fish & mussels

Instructions

Put ingredients in the slow cooker. Cover, and cook on low for 9 hours.

Bean Peppers stew

Serves 2

Ingredients - Allergies: SF, GF, DF, EF, NF

- 2 tbsp. coconut oil
- 1 onion, chopped
- 1 clove garlic, minced
- 3/4 pound minced pork meat
- 1/4 cup corn
- 1/4 cup tomato paste & 1/2 cups beef broth
- 1 tsp. cumin seeds & 1/4 tsp. ground cayenne pepper
- 1/4 tsp. salt
- 3/4 cup dry kidney beans
- 1 fresh hot chili pepper, chopped
- 1/4 cup chopped green and red pepper each

Instructions

Put ingredients in the slow cooker. Cover, and cook on low for 9 hours.

Pork Mushrooms stew

Serves 2

Ingredients - Allergies: SF, GF, DF, EF, NF

- 1 cup sliced mushrooms
- 1 chopped carrots
- 2 chopped onions
- 2 tbsp. coconut oil
- Salt, ground black pepper and ground cumin to taste
- 1 bay leaf & 1 Tsp. chopped garlic
- 1/2 cup beef stock & 2 Tsp. tomato paste
- 1 pound pork neck meat, cubed

Instructions

Put ingredients in the slow cooker. Cover, and cook on low for 9 hours.

Beef, Leeks & Cabbage stew

Serves 2

Ingredients - Allergies: SF, GF, DF, EF, NF

- 2 tbsp. coconut oil
- 3/4 cup leeks, chopped
- 1 clove garlic, minced
- 1 pound beef stew meat, cubed
- 1/2 cup beef broth
- 1 cup shredded cabbage
- 2 tsp. cumin seeds & 1/4 tsp. ground cayenne pepper
- 1/4 tsp. salt

Instructions

Put ingredients in the slow cooker. Cover, and cook on low for 9 hours.

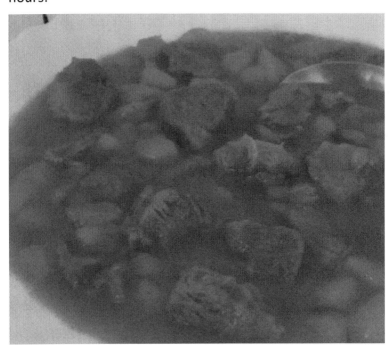

Chanko Nabe without Meatballs Sumo Stew

Serves 2

Ingredients - Allergies: SF, GF, DF, EF, NF

- 1/4 cup Shimeji and enoki mushrooms each (or shiitake)
- 1 Tbsp. dried seaweed
- Salt & 1/4 Tsp. ground pepper to taste
- 1 green onion, sliced
- 1 bok choy, sliced
- 1 carrot, sliced
- 1/2 cup napa cabbage, sliced
- 1 Tbsp. fish sauce
- 1 Tsp. miso paste (optional)
- 1 Tsp. minced ginger
- 1 cup fish broth
- 1/2 pounds thinly sliced pork
- 1/2 pounds shrimp

Instructions

Put ingredients in the slow cooker. Cover, and cook on low for 7 to 9 hours.

Beef, Parsnip & Turnip stew

Serves 2

Ingredients - Allergies: SF, GF, DF, EF, NF

- 2 tbsp. coconut oil
- 1/2 leek, chopped
- 1 clove garlic, minced
- 1 pound beef stewing meat
- 1/2 cups beef broth
- 2 tsp. cumin seeds & 1/4 tsp. ground cayenne pepper
- 1/4 tsp. salt
- 1/2 cups peeled and sliced parsnip
- 1 fresh hot chili peppers, chopped
- 1/4 cup peeled and sliced turnip

Instructions

Put ingredients in the slow cooker. Cover, and cook on low for 9 hours.

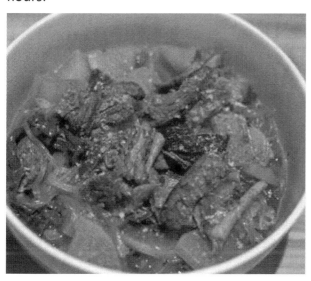

Mongolian Spicy Beef stew

Serves 2

Ingredients - Allergies: SF, GF, DF, EF, NF

- 2 tbsp. coconut oil
- 1 onion, chopped
- 1 clove garlic, minced
- 1 pound flanked steak
- 1/4 cup tomato paste & 1/4 cups beef broth
- 2 tsp. cumin seeds & 1/4 tsp. ground cayenne pepper
- 1/4 tsp. salt
- 1 cup celery
- 1 fresh hot chili peppers, chopped
- 1 chopped green onion

Instructions

Put ingredients in the slow cooker. Cover, and cook on low for 9 hours.

Pork & White Beans stew

Serves 2

Ingredients - Allergies: SF, GF, DF, EF, NF

- 2 tbsp. coconut oil
- 1 red onion, chopped
- 1 clove garlic, minced
- 3/4 pound minced pork meat
- 1 tomato & 1/2 cup beef broth
- 1 tsp. cumin seeds & 1/4 tsp. ground cayenne pepper
- 1/4 tsp. salt
- 3/4 cups dry white beans
- 1 fresh hot chili peppers, chopped
- 1/2 cup chopped celery

Instructions

Put ingredients in the slow cooker. Cover, and cook on low for 9 hours.

Green Beans & Chicken stew

Serves 2

Ingredients - Allergies: SF, GF, DF, EF, NF

- 2 tbsp. coconut oil
- 1 onions, chopped
- 1 clove garlic, minced
- 1 pound chicken meat
- 1/2 cup chicken broth
- 1/4 tsp. cumin seeds & 1/4 tsp. ground cayenne pepper
- 1/4 tsp. salt
- 1 cup green beans
- 1 small chopped tomato
- 1/2 cups chopped celery

Instructions

Put ingredients in the slow cooker. Cover, and cook on low for 9 hours.

Bulgarian Chicken stew

Serves 2

Ingredients - Allergies: SF, GF, DF, EF, NF

- 2 tbsp. coconut oil
- 1 onion, chopped
- 1 clove garlic, minced
- 1 pound dark chicken meat
- 1/4 cup tomato paste & 1/2 cups chicken broth
- 1/4 tsp. ground cayenne pepper
- 1/4 tsp. salt
- 1 carrot and 1 turnip, sliced
- 3/4 cups chopped celery

Instructions

Put ingredients in the slow cooker. Cover, and cook on low for 9 hours.

3 Beans Chili

Serves 2

Ingredients - Allergies: SF, GF, DF, EF, NF

- 2 tbsp. <u>coconut</u> oil
- 1 onion, chopped
- 3 clove garlic, minced
- 1/4 pound ground beef
- 1/4 pound beef sirloin, cubed
- 1/2 cup diced tomatoes
- 1 cup beef broth
- 1 tsp. cumin seeds
- 1/4 tsp. dried oregano
- 1/4 tsp. ground cayenne pepper
- 1/4 tsp. ground coriander
- 1/4 tsp. salt
- 1/4 cup dry kidney beans
- 1/4 cup dry navy beans
- 1/4 cup dry navy beans
- 1/4 fresh hot chili peppers, chopped

Instructions

Put ingredients in the slow cooker. Cover, and cook on low for 9 hours.

Pork & Liver stew

Serves 2

Ingredients - Allergies: SF, GF, DF, EF, NF

- 2 tbsp. coconut oil
- 1 onion, chopped
- 1 clove garlic, minced
- 1/2 pound pork neck meat
- 1/4 cup tomato paste & 1/2 cup beef broth
- 1/4 tsp. cumin seeds & 1/4 tsp. ground cayenne pepper
- 1/4 tsp. salt
- 1/2 pound veal liver, cubed
- 1 fresh hot chili peppers, chopped
- 1 cups chopped celery

Instructions

Put ingredients in the slow cooker. Cover, and cook on low for 9 hours.

Pork Tenderloin stew

Serves 2

Ingredients - Allergies: SF, GF, DF, EF, NF

- 2 tbsp. coconut oil
- 1 onion, chopped
- 1 clove garlic, minced
- 1 pound pork tenderloin meat
- 1/2 cups beef broth
- 1 tsp. cumin seeds & 1/4 tsp. ground cayenne pepper
- 1/4 tsp. salt
- 1 cup mushrooms, sliced
- 1 carrot, chopped
- 1 cup chopped celery

Instructions

Put ingredients in the slow cooker. Cover, and cook on low for 9 hours.

Chicken Onion Celery Stew

Serves 2

Ingredients - Allergies: SF, GF, DF, EF, NF

- 2 tbsp. coconut oil
- 1 small onion, chopped
- 1 clove garlic, minced
- 1 pound dark chicken meat
- 1/2 cups beef broth
- 1/2 tsp. cumin seeds & 1/4 tsp. ground cayenne pepper
- 1/4 tsp. salt
- 2 cups chopped celery

Instructions

Put ingredients in the slow cooker. Cover, and cook on low for 9 hours.

Goulash Soup

Serves 2

Ingredients - Allergies: SF, GF, DF, EF, NF

- 2 tbsp. coconut oil
- 1 small onion, chopped
- 1 clove garlic, minced
- 1 pound beef stew meat
- 2 cups beef broth
- 1/2 tsp. cumin seeds & 1/4 tsp. ground cayenne pepper
- 1 tsp. ground red paprika
- 1/4 tsp. salt
- 1 small carrot, chopped
- 1 cup chopped celery

Instructions

Put ingredients in the slow cooker. Cover, and cook on low for 9 hours.

Pork Veal stew

Serves 2

Ingredients - Allergies: SF, GF, DF, EF, NF

- 2 tbsp. coconut oil
- 1 small onion, chopped
- 1 clove garlic, minced
- 1/2 pound pork and veal stew meat each
- 1/2 cup beef broth
- 1/2 tsp. cumin seeds & 1/4 tsp. ground cayenne pepper
- 1/4 tsp. salt
- 1 cup mushrooms, sliced
- 1 small carrot, chopped
- 1 cup chopped celery

Instructions

Put ingredients in the slow cooker. Cover, and cook on low for 9 hours.

Venison Portobello Mushroom stew

Serves 2

Ingredients - Allergies: SF, GF, DF, EF, NF

- 2 tbsp. coconut oil
- 1 small onion, chopped
- 1 clove garlic, minced
- 1 pound venison meat
- 1/4 cup beef broth
- 1/2 tsp. cumin seeds & 1/4 tsp. ground cayenne pepper
- 1/4 tsp. salt
- 1/2 cups Portobello mushrooms, sliced
- 1 small carrot, chopped
- 1 cups chopped celery

Instructions

Put ingredients in the slow cooker. Cover, and cook on low for 9 hours.

Venison Celery stew

Serves 2

Ingredients - Allergies: SF, GF, DF, EF, NF

- 2 tbsp. coconut oil
- 1 small onion, chopped
- 1 clove garlic, minced
- 1 pound venison meat
- 1/4 cup beef broth
- 1/2 tsp. cumin seeds & 1/4 tsp. ground cayenne pepper
- 1/4 tsp. salt
- 1 small carrot, chopped
- 2 cups chopped celery

Instructions

Put ingredients in the slow cooker. Cover, and cook on low for 9 hours.

Stir Fries

Pork and Bok Choy / Celery Stir Fry
Allergies: SF, GF, DF, EF, NF

10 oz. Lean Pork Tenderloin and 2 cups Bok Choy / Celery stir fry. Use as much veggies as you want or replace Bok Choy with Kale. Season with fish sauce.

Lemon Chicken Stir Fry

Ingredients - Allergies: SF, GF, DF, EF, NF

- 1/2 lemon
- 1/4 cup chicken broth
- 1 tbsp. fish sauce
- 1 teaspoons arrowroot flour
- 1/2 tbsp. coconut oil
- 1/2 pound boneless, skinless chicken breasts, trimmed and cut into 1-inch pieces
- 5 ounces mushrooms, halved or quartered
- 1 cup snow peas, stems and strings removed
- 1 bunch scallions, cut into 1-inch pieces, white and green parts divided
- 1 tbsp. chopped garlic

Instructions

Grate 1 tsp. lemon zest. Juice the lemon and mix 3 tbsp. of the juice with broth, fish sauce and arrowroot flour in a small bowl.

Heat oil in a skillet over high heat. Add chicken and cook, stirring occasionally, until just cooked through. Transfer to a plate. Add mushrooms to the pan and cook until the mushrooms are tender. Add snow peas, garlic, scallion whites and the lemon zest. Cook, stirring, around 30 seconds. Add the broth to the pan and cook, stirring, 2 to 3 minutes. Add scallion greens and the chicken and any accumulated juices and stir.

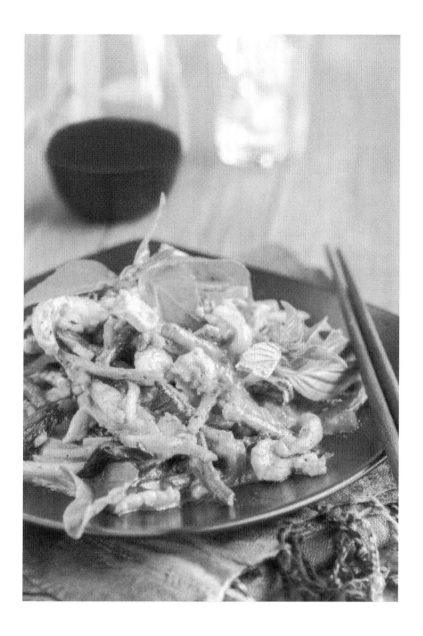

Pan seared Brussels sprouts

Serves 2

Ingredients - Allergies: SF, GF, DF, EF, NF

- 6 oz. cubed pork
- 2 tbsp. <u>coconut oil</u>
- 1 pound Brussels sprouts, halved
- 1/2 large onion, chopped
- Salt and ground black pepper

Instructions

Cook pork in a skillet over high heat. Remove to a plate and chop. In same pan with pork fat, add coconut oil over high heat. Add onions and Brussels sprouts and cook, stirring occasionally, until sprouts are golden brown. Season with salt and pepper, to taste, and put pork back into pan. Serve immediately.

Beef and Broccoli Stir Fry

Allergies: SF, GF, DF, EF, NF

• 10 oz. of lean Beef and 2 cups broccoli stir fry. Use as much broccoli as you want or replace Broccoli with Kale.

Garbanzo Stir Fry

Serves 2

Ingredients - Allergies: SF, GF, DF, EF, V, NF

- 2 tbsp. coconut oil
- 1 tbsp. oregano
- 1 tbsp. chopped basil
- 1 clove garlic, crushed
- ground black pepper to taste
- 2 cups cooked garbanzo beans

- 1 large zucchini, halved and sliced
- 1/2 cup sliced mushrooms
- 1 tbsp. chopped cilantro
- 1 tomato, chopped

Heat oil in a skillet over medium heat. Stir in oregano, basil, garlic and pepper. Add the garbanzo beans and zucchini, stirring well to coat with oil and herbs. Cook for 10 minutes, stirring occasionally. Stir in mushrooms and cilantro; cook 10 minutes, stirring occasionally. Place the chopped tomato on top of the mixture to steam. Cover and cook 5 minutes more.

Thai Basil Chicken

Ingredients - Allergies: SF, GF, DF, NF

Eggs

- 2 eggs
- 2 tbsp. of <u>coconut oil</u> for frying

Basil chicken

- 2 chicken breast (or any other cut of boneless chicken)
- 5 cloves of garlic
- 4 Thai chilies
- 1 tbsp. coconut oil for frying
- Fish sauce
- 1 handful of Thai holy basil leaves

Instructions

First, fry the eggs

Basil chicken

Cut the chicken into small pieces. Peel the garlic and chilies, and chop them fine. Add basil leaves.

Add about 1 tbsp. of oil to the pan.

When the oil is hot, add the chilies and garlic. Stir fry for half a minute.

Toss in your chicken and keep stir frying. Add fish sauce.

Add basil into the pan, fold it into the chicken, and turn off the heat.

Shrimp with Snow Peas

Ingredients - Allergies: SF, GF, DF, EF, NF

Marinade

- 1 teaspoon arrowroot flour
- 1 Tbsp. wine
- 1/4 tsp. salt

Stir Fry

- 1/2 pound shrimp. Peel the shrimp and take the vein out
- 1 Tbsp coconut oil
- 1/2 Tbsp minced ginger
- 1 garlic cloves, sliced thinly
- 1 cup snow peas, strings removed
- 1 teaspoons fish sauce
- 1/4 cup chicken broth
- 2 green onions, white and light green parts, sliced diagonally
- 1 teaspoons dark roasted sesame oil

Instructions

Mix all the ingredients for the marinade in a bowl and then add the shrimp. Mix to coat. Let it marinade 15 minutes while you prepare the peas, ginger, and garlic.

Add the coconut oil in the wok and let it get hot. Add the garlic and ginger and combine. Stir-fry for about 30 seconds.

Add the marinade to the wok, add the snow peas, fish sauce and chicken broth. Stir-fry until the shrimp turns pink. Add the green onions and stir-fry for one more minute. Turn off the heat and add the sesame oil.

Pork and Green Beans Stir Fry

Allergies: SF, GF, DF, EF, NF

- 10 oz. of lean Pork

- 2 cups of Green Beans, snapped in half. Use as much veggies as you want or replace Green beans with Kale.

- 2 garlic clove, chopped

- 1 inch of peeled and chopped ginger

- Season with fish sauce.

Cashew chicken

Ingredients - Allergies: SF, GF, DF, EF, NF

- 1/2 bunch scallions
- 1/2 pound skinless boneless chicken thighs
- 1/4 tsp. salt
- 1/8 tsp. black pepper
- 2 tbsp. coconut oil
- 1/2 red bell pepper and 1 stalk of celery, chopped
- 2 garlic cloves, finely chopped
- 1 tbsp. finely chopped peeled fresh ginger
- 1/8 tsp. dried hot red-pepper flakes
- 1/4 cup chicken broth
- 1 tbsp. fish sauce
- 1 teaspoons arrowroot flour
- 1/4 cup salted roasted whole cashews

Instructions

Chop scallions and separate green and white parts. Pat chicken dry and cut into 3/4-inch pieces and season with salt and pepper. Heat a wok or a skillet over high heat. Add oil and then stir-fry chicken until cooked through, 3 to 4 minutes. Transfer to a plate. Add garlic, bell pepper, celery, ginger, red-pepper flakes, and scallion whites to wok and stir-fry until peppers are just tender, 4 to 5 minutes.

Mix together broth, fish sauce and arrowroot flour, then stir into vegetables in wok. Reduce heat and simmer, stirring occasionally, until thickened. Stir in cashews, scallion greens, and chicken along with any juices.

Mushrooms, Snow Peas & Bok Choy Stir Fry

Serves 2

Ingredients - Allergies: SF, GF, DF, EF

- 1/2 pound mushrooms
- 1 cup Snow Peas
- 1 cup sliced Bok Choy
- 1/2 cup sliced onions
- 1 Tsp. coconut oil

Instructions

Marinade mushrooms in a Superfoods marinade. Stir fry drained mushrooms in coconut oil for few minutes, add onions and Snow Peas and stir fry for 2 more minutes. Add the rest of the marinade and bok choy and stir fry for a minute. Serve with brown rice or quinoa.

Pork, Red Peppers, Carrots, Celery & Basil Stir Fry
Serves 2

Ingredients - Allergies: SF, GF, DF, EF

- 1/2 pound cubed pork
- 1 cup sliced Red Peppers
- 1/2 cup sliced celery
- 1/2 cup sliced carrots
- 1 Tsp. coconut oil
- 2 Tbsp. sliced Basil leaves

Instructions

Marinade pork in a Superfoods marinade. Stir fry drained pork in coconut oil for few minutes, add carrots and celery and stir fry for 2 more minutes. Add the rest of the marinade and basil leaves and stir fry for a minute. Serve with brown rice or quinoa.

Pork, Zucchini & Onions Stir Fry

Serves 2

Ingredients - Allergies: SF, GF, DF, EF

- 1/2 pound pork
- 1 cup sliced Zucchini
- 1 cup sliced onions
- 1 Tsp. coconut oil

Instructions

Marinade pork in a Superfoods marinade. Stir fry drained pork in coconut oil for few minutes, add zucchini and onions and stir fry for 2 more minutes. Add the rest of the marinade and stir fry for a minute. Serve with brown rice or quinoa.

Snow Peas, Shrimp, Mushrooms & Bok Choy Stir Fry
Serves 2

Ingredients - Allergies: SF, GF, DF, EF

- 1/2 pound shrimp
- 1 cup sliced Snow peas
- 1 cup sliced Chinese celery
- 1/2 cup sliced mushrooms
- 1 Tsp. coconut oil

Instructions

Marinade shrimp in a Superfoods marinade. Stir fry drained shrimp in coconut oil for few minutes, add snow peas and Chinese celery and stir fry for 2 more minutes. Add the rest of the marinade and mushrooms and stir fry for a minute. Serve with brown rice or quinoa.

Eggplant, Red Peppers & Carrots Stir Fry

Serves 2

Ingredients - Allergies: SF, GF, DF, EF

- 1/2 pound Red Peppers
- 1 + 1/2 cup sliced Eggplant
- 1 cup sliced Carrots
- 1/2 cup sliced onions
- 1 Tsp. coconut oil

Instructions

Marinade eggplant in a Superfoods marinade. Stir fry drained eggplant and carrots in coconut oil for 5 minutes, add red peppers and onions, stir fry for 2 more minutes. Add the rest of the marinade and stir fry for a minute. Serve with brown rice or quinoa.

Eggplant, Shiitake & Bamboo Shoots Stir Fry

Serves 2

Ingredients - Allergies: SF, GF, DF, EF

- 1/2 pound sliced shiitake mushrooms
- 1 cup sliced eggplant
- 1 cup sliced Green peppers
- 1/2 cup sliced carrots
- 1/2 cup sliced onions
- 1/2 cup sliced bamboo shoots
- 1 Tsp. coconut oil

Instructions

Marinade shiitake, bamboo shoots and eggplant in a Superfoods marinade. Stir fry drained eggplant and bamboo shoots in coconut oil for 5 minutes, add carrots and onions and stir fry for 2 more minutes. Add the rest of the marinade with shiitake and stir fry for a minute. Serve with brown rice or quinoa.

Korean Squid Stir Fry
Serves 2

Ingredients - Allergies: SF, GF, DF, EF

- 1 pound Squid stripes
- 1 cup sliced carrots
- 1/2 cup Korean Spicy marinade
- 1/2 cup sliced onions
- 1 Tsp. coconut oil

Instructions

Marinade squid stripes in a Korean spicy marinade. Stir fry drained squid in coconut oil for few minutes, add carrots and onions and stir fry for 2 more minutes. Add the rest of the marinade and stir fry for a minute. Serve with brown rice or quinoa.

Okra, Sprouts & Onions Choy Stir Fry

Serves 2

Ingredients - Allergies: SF, GF, DF, EF

- 1 + 1/2 pound sliced okra
- 1 cup sprouts
- 1/2 cup sliced onions
- 1 Tsp. coconut oil

Instructions

Marinade okra in a Superfoods marinade. Stir fry drained okra in coconut oil for few minutes, add onions and stir fry for 2 more minutes. Add the rest of the marinade and sprouts and stir fry for a minute. Serve with brown rice or quinoa.

Okra, Asparagus, Chicken & Onions Stir Fry

Serves 2

Ingredients - Allergies: SF, GF, DF, EF

- 1/2 pound chicken
- 1 cup sliced okra
- 1 cup sliced asparagus
- 1/2 cup sliced onions
- 1 Tsp. coconut oil

Instructions

Marinade chicken in a Korean Spicy marinade. Stir fry drained chicken in coconut oil for few minutes, add okra and asparagus and stir fry for 2 more minutes. Add the rest of the marinade and onions and stir fry for a minute. Serve with brown rice or quinoa.

Okra, Ground Beef, Red Peppers & Cilantro Stir Fry
Serves 2

Ingredients - Allergies: SF, GF, DF, EF

- 1/2 pound ground beef
- 1 cup sliced okra
- 1 cup sliced red peppers
- 1/2 cup sliced onions
- 1/4 cup sliced cilantro
- 1 Tsp. coconut oil

Instructions
Marinade okra in a Superfoods marinade. Stir fry drained okra and ground beef in coconut oil for few minutes, add red peppers and onions and stir fry for 2 more minutes. Add the rest of the marinade and half of cilantro and stir fry for a minute. Decorate with the rest of cilantro. Serve with brown rice or quinoa.

Pork, Broccoli, Baby Carrots & Mushrooms Stir Fry

Serves 2

Ingredients - Allergies: SF, GF, DF, EF

- 1/2 pound cubed pork
- 1 cup sliced Broccoli
- 1 cup halved lengthwise baby carrots
- 1/2 cup sliced mushrooms
- 1 Tsp. coconut oil

Instructions

Marinade pork in a Superfoods marinade. Stir fry drained pork in coconut oil for few minutes, add broccoli and baby carrots and stir fry for 2 more minutes. Add the rest of the marinade and mushrooms and stir fry for a minute. Serve with brown rice or quinoa.

Pork, Red Peppers, Broccoli & Carrots Stir Fry

Serves 2

Ingredients - Allergies: SF, GF, DF, EF

- 1/2 pound pork
- 1 cup sliced Red Peppers
- 1 cup sliced Broccoli
- 1/2 cup sliced carrots
- 1 Tsp. coconut oil

Instructions

Marinade pork in a Superfoods marinade. Stir fry drained pork in coconut oil for few minutes, add broccoli and carrots and stir fry for 2 more minutes. Add the rest of the marinade and red peppers and stir fry for a minute. Serve with brown rice or quinoa.

Green Peas, Pork, Onions & Cilntro Stir Fry
Serves 2

Ingredients - Allergies: SF, GF, DF, EF

- 1/2 pound pork
- 1 cup Green peas
- 1 cup sliced onions
- 1/4 cup cilantro
- 1 Tsp. coconut oil

Instructions
Marinade pork in a Superfoods marinade. Stir fry drained pork and green peas in coconut oil for few minutes, add onions and stir fry for 2 more minutes. Add the rest of the marinade and stir fry for a minute. Serve with brown rice or quinoa.

Bitter Gourd, Shrimp & Squid Stir Fry
Serves 2

Ingredients - Allergies: SF, GF, DF, EF

- 1/2 pound squid slices
- 1/2 pound shrimp
- 1 cup sliced bitter gourd
- 1/2 cup sliced onions
- 1 Tsp. coconut oil

Instructions

Marinade shrimp and squid in a Superfoods marinade. Stir fry drained shrimp and squid in coconut oil for few minutes, add bitter gourd and stir fry for 2 more minutes. Add the rest of the marinade and onions and stir fry for a minute. Serve with brown rice or quinoa.

Baby Carrots & Shrimp Stir Fry
Serves 2

Ingredients - Allergies: SF, GF, DF, EF

- 1/2 pound shrimp
- 1 cup baby carrots
- 1/2 cup sliced Broccoli
- 1/2 cup sliced mushrooms
- 1 Tsp. coconut oil

Instructions

Marinade pork in a Superfoods marinade. Stir fry drained shrimp in coconut oil for few minutes, add broccoli and carrots and stir fry for 2 more minutes. Add the rest of the marinade and mushrooms and stir fry for a minute. Serve with brown rice or quinoa.

Beef, Onions & Chili Stir Fry

Serves 2

Ingredients - Allergies: SF, GF, DF, EF

- 1/2 pound beef
- 1 cup sliced onions
- 1/2 cup sliced celery
- 1 Tsp. coconut oil
- 1 Tsp. chili sauce (to taste)

Instructions

Marinade pork in a Superfoods marinade with chili sauce added. Stir fry drained beef in coconut oil for few minutes, add onions and celery and stir fry for 2 more minutes. Add the rest of the marinade and red peppers and stir fry for a minute. Serve with brown rice or quinoa.

Black Pepper Beef & Green Peppers Stir Fry
Serves 2

Ingredients - Allergies: SF, GF, DF, EF

- 1/2 pound beef
- 1 cup sliced Green Peppers
- 1 cup sliced Onion
- 1/2 cup sliced celery
- 1 Tbsp. coconut oil

Instructions
Marinade beef in a Superfoods marinade. Stir fry drained beef in coconut oil for few minutes, add celery and onions and stir fry for 2 more minutes. Add the rest of the marinade and green peppers and stir fry for a minute. Serve with brown rice or quinoa.

Lamb, Mushrooms & Broccoli Stir Fry

Serves 2

Ingredients - Allergies: SF, GF, DF, EF

- 1/2 pound lamb
- 1 cup sliced Mushrooms
- 1 cup sliced Broccoli
- 1/2 cup sliced onions
- 1 Tbsp. coconut oil

Instructions

Marinade lamb in a Superfoods marinade. Stir fry drained lamb in coconut oil for few minutes, add broccoli and onions and stir fry for 2 more minutes. Add the rest of the marinade and mushrooms and stir fry for a minute. Serve with brown rice or quinoa.

Pork, Carrots & Spinach Stir Fry

Serves 2

Ingredients - Allergies: SF, GF, DF, EF

- 1/2 pound pork
- 1 cup spinach
- 1 cup sliced carrots
- 1 Tbsp. coconut oil

Instructions

Marinade pork in a Superfoods marinade. Stir fry drained pork in coconut oil for few minutes, add carrots and stir fry for 2 more minutes. Add the rest of the marinade and spinach and stir fry for a minute. Serve with brown rice or quinoa.

Pork, Bok Choy & GreenPeppers Stir Fry
Serves 2

Ingredients - Allergies: SF, GF, DF, EF

- 1/2 pound pork
- 1 cup sliced Green Peppers
- 1 cup sliced Bok Choy
- 1/2 cup sliced green onions
- 1 Tbsp. coconut oil

Instructions

Marinade pork in a Superfoods marinade. Stir fry drained pork in coconut oil for few minutes, add white parts of bok choy and green onions and stir fry for 2 more minutes. Add the rest of the marinade and green peppers and the rest of bok choy and stir fry for a minute. Serve with brown rice or quinoa.

Pork, Green Onions & Red Peppers Stir Fry

Serves 2

Ingredients - Allergies: SF, GF, DF, EF

- 1/2 pound pork
- 1 cup sliced Red Peppers
- 1 cup sliced green onions
- 1/2 cup sliced carrots
- 1 Tbsp. coconut oil

Instructions

Marinade pork in a Superfoods marinade. Stir fry drained pork in coconut oil for few minutes, add green onions and carrots and stir fry for 2 more minutes. Add the rest of the marinade and red peppers and stir fry for a minute. Serve with brown rice or quinoa.

Meats

Baked Chicken Breast with Fresh Basil

Ingredients - Allergies: SF, GF, EF, NF

- 2 boneless skinless chicken breast
- 1/4 cup low-fat yogurt
- 1/4 cup chopped basil
- 1 tsp. arrowroot flour
- 2 Tbsp. oatmeal, coarsely ground

Instructions

Arrange chicken in a baking dish. Combine basil, yogurt and arrowroot flour; mix well and spread over chicken.

Mix oatmeal with salt and pepper to taste and sprinkle over chicken.

Bake chicken in 375 degrees in the oven for half an hour.

Roast Chicken with Rosemary

- 2 chicken pieces, skinned
- salt and pepper to taste
- 1 onion, quartered
- 2 Tbsp. chopped rosemary

Instructions - Allergies: SF, GF, DF, EF, NF

Heat the oven to 350F. Sprinkle meat with salt and pepper. Cover with the onion and rosemary. Place in a baking dish and bake in the preheated oven until chicken is cooked through.

Carne Asada

Allergies: SF, GF, DF, EF, NF

Marinade:

Mix together the garlic, jalapeno, cilantro, salt, and pepper to make a paste. Put the paste in a container. Add the oil and lime juice. Shake it up to combine. Use as a marinade for beef or as a table condiment.

Instructions

Put the 1 pound flank steak in a baking dish and pour the marinade over it. Refrigerate up to 8 hours.

Take the steak out of the marinade and season it on both sides with salt and pepper. Grill (or broil) the steak for 7 to 10 minutes per side, turning once, until medium-rare. Put the steak on a cutting board and allow the juices to settle (5 minutes). Thinly slice the steak across the grain.

Meatballs

Baked Beef Meatballs

Allergies: SF, GF, NF

- 1/2 pound lean ground beef
- 1 tbsp. minced onion
- 1/4 tsp. minced garlic
- 1/2 tsp. parmesan cheese
- 1 egg
- 1/4 tsp. salt
- 1/8 tsp. pepper

Mix all of the ingredients in a large bowl using your fingers. Mix until the meat no long feels slimy from the eggs. Shape in small egg size meatballs. Place on a baking sheet. Bake at 375F for 20-25 minutes until the meatballs are cooked through. Serve with large Fiber Loaded salad with Italian Dressing.

Middle Eastern Meatballs

Allergies: SF, GF, DF, EF, NF

Ingredients

- 1 pound ground lamb or beef, or a mixture of the two
- 1/2 Onion, minced
- 1/4 of a bunch of fresh parsley or mint, finely chopped
- Ground cumin – 1/2 tbsp.
- Cinnamon -- 1 teaspoons
- Allspice (optional) – 1/2 tsp.
- Salt and pepper -- to season
- Coconut Oil – 2 Tbsp.

Instructions

Place the ground beef or lamb, onion, herbs, spices, salt and pepper in a bowl and knead well. Chill for 1-2 hours and let the flavors mingle. Form the meat into patties or balls the size of a small egg.

Bake in the oven on 350F. Serve with tzatziki sauce.

Variations

Experiment with different seasonings--coriander, cayenne, sesame seeds.

Casseroles

Broccoli Chicken Casserole

Ingredients - Allergies: SF, GF, NF

- 2 cups broccoli florets
- 10 oz. skinless, boneless chicken (or turkey) pieces (breast or dark meat)
- 2 tsp of <u>flax</u> seeds meal
- Salt, pepper
- 2 eggs - beaten
- 1 cup of Yogurt Dressing (or coconut milk, if you don't like the sourish tang)
- 1/2 cup of chicken broth
- 4 tbsp. of grated low-fat cheddar cheese

Heat the oven to 400°. Cook broccoli around 5 minutes. Take broccoli out and add chicken (or turkey) and simmer for 15 minutes. Cut chicken (or turkey) into cubes and add it to the broccoli.

Combine broth, flax, salt and pepper in a pan and mix. Bring to a boil over high heat and cook 1 minute, stirring constantly. Remove from heat. Add yogurt dressing, beaten egg and then half of the cheese, stirring until well combined. Add sauce to broccoli mixture; and stir gently until combined.

Put mixture in a small casserole dish oiled with some coconut oil. Put remaining cheese on top, sprinkle. Bake at 400° for 50 minutes or until mixture bubbles at the edges and cheese begins to brown. Remove from oven and let cool for 5 minutes.

Beef Meatballs Broccoli Casserole

Ingredients - Allergies: SF, GF

- 2 cups broccoli florets
- 10 oz. beef meatballs (see separate recipe)
- 2 tsp of almond flour
- Salt, pepper
- 2 eggs - beaten
- 1 cup of Yogurt Dressing
- 1/2 cup of chicken broth
- 2 tbsp. of grated low-fat cheddar cheese

Instructions

Heat oven to 400F. Cook broccoli around 5 minutes. Prepare beef meatballs as in the recipe above. Combine broth, flour, salt and pepper in a saucepan, stirring with a whisk until smooth. Bring to a boil over medium-high heat; cook 1 minute, stirring constantly. Remove from heat. Add yogurt dressing, beaten egg and then half of the cheese, stirring until well combined. Add sauce to broccoli mixture; and stir gently until combined.
Put mixture in a small casserole dish oiled with some coconut oil. Sprinkle with remaining cheese. Bake at 400° for 50 minutes or until mixture bubbles at the edges and cheese begins to brown. Remove from oven and let cool for 5 minutes. Serve with large Fiber Loaded Salad with Italian Dressing.

Beef Meatballs Cauliflower Casserole

Ingredients - Allergies: SF, GF

- 2 cups cauliflower florets
- 10 oz. beef meatballs (see separate recipe)
- 2 tsp of almond flour
- Salt, pepper
- 2 eggs - beaten
- 1 cup of Yogurt Dressing
- 1/2 cup of chicken broth
- 2 tbsp of grated low-fat cheddar cheese

Instructions

Heat oven to 400°.
Cook cauliflower around 5 minutes. Prepare beef meatballs as in the recipe above. Combine soup, flour, salt and pepper in a saucepan, stirring with a whisk until smooth. Bring to a boil over medium-high heat; cook 1 minute, stirring constantly. Remove from heat. Add yogurt dressing, beaten egg and then half of the cheese, stirring until well combined. Add sauce to cauliflower mixture; and stir gently until combined.
Put mixture in a small casserole dish oiled with some coconut oil. Sprinkle with remaining cheese. Bake at 400° for 50 minutes or until mixture bubbles at the edges and cheese begins to brown. Remove from oven and let cool for 5 minutes. Serve with large Fiber Loaded Salad with Italian Dressing.

Cabbage Roll Casserole

Ingredients - Allergies: SF, GF, DF, EF, NF

1/2 pounds ground beef
1/4 cup chopped onion
1 cup tomato sauce
1 pound cabbage or sauerkraut leaves
1/4 cup uncooked brown rice
1/4 tsp. salt
1/2 cup beef broth

Instructions

Heat oven to 350F.
Brown beef in coconut oil in a skillet over medium high heat until through. In a large mixing bowl combine the onion, rice and salt. Add meat and mix all together. Roll mixture into cabbage leaves and arrange them in a casserole dish. Pour broth and tomato sauce over rolls and bake in the preheated oven, covered, for 1 hour.

Chia, Flax & Broccoli Casserole

Serves 2

Ingredients - Allergies: SF, GF, DF, EF, NF

- 1 cup broccoli florets
- 1 small chopped onion
- 1 tbsp. coconut oil
- 1 cup healthy casserole sour cream
- 1/4 cup flax seeds meal
- 1/4 cup chia seeds

Instructions

Put broccoli and onion in the casserole dish, mix sauce, flax and chia seeds, pour sauce on top, cover and bake for 1 1/2 hours on 400F.

Slow cooked Sweet Potatoes & Tomato Casserole

Serves 2

Ingredients - Allergies: SF, GF, DF, EF, NF

- 1 cup chopped sweet potatoes
- 1 large chopped onions
- 1 tbsp. coconut oil
- 1 cup sliced tomatoes
- 1 cup healthy casserole sour cream
- 1 Tbsp. chopped parsley

Instructions

Put all recipe ingredients in the casserole dish, pour sauce on top, arrange sliced tomatoes on top, cover and bake for 2 hours on 400F. Garnish with parsley.

Eggplant, Zucchini and Tomato Casserole
Serves 8

Ingredients - Allergies: SF, GF, DF, EF, NF

- 1-1/2 cups sliced zucchini
- 1-1/2 cups sliced tomatoes
- 2 tbsp. coconut oil
- 1-1/2 cups sliced eggplant
- 1/2 tsp. salt
- 1/4 tsp. ground black pepper
- 1/2 tsp. minced garlic

Instructions

Arrange all ingredients in the casserole dish (see picture), cover and bake for 1 1-2 hours on 400F.

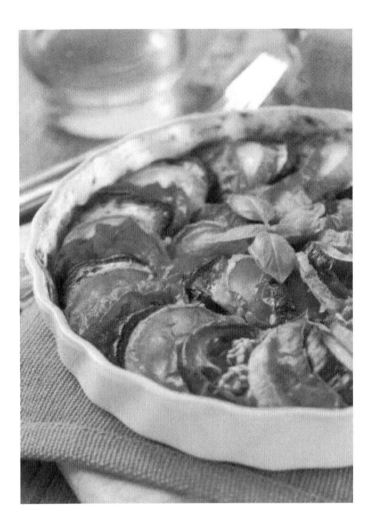

Zucchini & Chicken Casserole

Serves 8

Ingredients - Allergies: SF, GF, DF, EF, NF

- 1-1/2 cups sliced zucchini
- 1 cup chopped onions
- 2 tbsp. <u>coconut</u> oil
- 2 tbsp. chopped green onions
- 1 cup healthy casserole sauce

Instructions

Put ingredients in the casserole dish, pour sauce on top, cover and bake for 1 1/2 hours on 400F. Sprinkle with green onions before serving..

Red Peppers, Zucchini and Eggplant Casserole

Serves 8

Ingredients - Allergies: SF, GF, DF, EF, NF

- 2 chopped carrots
- 1 - 1/2 cup chopped onions
- 1 - 1/2 cup sliced red peppers
- 4 tbsp. coconut oil
- 1 cup sliced zucchini
- 1/2 tsp. salt
- 1/4 tsp. ground black pepper
- 1/2 tsp. minced garlic
- 1/2 tsp. oregano
- 2 pounds sliced eggplant
- 1 cup Tomato Paste

Instructions

Put all recipe ingredients in the casserole dish, cover and bake for 2 hours on 400F.

Pork Chop Casserole

Ingredients - Allergies: SF, GF, DF, EF, NF

- 1/2 cup vegetable broth
- 1/4 cup brown rice
- 4 ounce mushrooms
- salt and pepper to taste
- 2 thick pork chops

Instructions

Heat oven to 350F. Pour broth into a baking dish. Add rice and mushrooms and mix. Salt and pepper to taste. Add pork chops in a single layer on that mixture and push them down into mixture and make sure they are covered with it.

Cover baking dish with aluminum foil and bake for 1 hour.

Mushrooms Casserole

Instructions – Allergies: SF, GF, NF

- 1 1/2 pounds sliced mushrooms (shiitake preferably)
- 1/2 pound sliced leeks
- Salt and freshly ground black pepper
- 1/2 tbsp. chopped parsley
- 1 beaten egg
- 1/2 cup of low-fat Greek yogurt
- 1/4 cup of shredded cheddar cheese, low-fat
- 1/2 pound cubed skinless boneless chicken (or turkey) breasts

Instructions

Heat oven to 375 degrees F. Mix beaten eggs and low-fat yogurt in a separate dish. In a casserole, place 1 layer of mushrooms, leeks and chicken cubes and season with salt, pepper, and parsley. Cover with 1/2 of a cup of eggs/yogurt mixture. Repeat process 2 more times and cover with shredded cheese. Bake until mushrooms and chicken is tender and crust is golden brown. Serve with Large Fiber Loaded salad with Italian Dressing.

Chicken Eggplant Casserole

Ingredients – Allergies: SF, GF, NF

- 1 pound Eggplant
- Salt and ground black pepper
- 1/2 tbsp. chopped parsley
- 1 beaten eggs
- 1/2 cup of low-fat Greek yogurt
- 1/4 cup of shredded cheddar cheese, low-fat
- 1/2 pound cubed skinless boneless chicken (or turkey) breasts

Instructions

Preheat oven to 375 degrees F. Mix beaten eggs and low-fat yogurt in a separate dish. In a casserole, place 1 layer of eggplant and meat cubes. Sprinkle with salt, pepper, and parsley. Cover with 1/2 of a cup of eggs/yogurt mixture. Repeat process 2 more times and cover with shredded cheese. Bake until eggplant and chicken are tender and crust is golden brown, about 20 minutes. Serve with Large Fiber Loaded salad with Italian Dressing.

Beef Meatballs Green Beans Casserole

Ingredients - Allergies: SF, GF

- 2 cups green beans florets
- 10 oz. beef meatballs (see separate recipe)
- 2 tsp of <u>almond</u> flour
- Salt, pepper
- 3 eggs - beaten

Half a cup of Yogurt Dressing

- 1/2 cup of chicken broth
- 4 tbsp. of grated low-fat cheddar cheese

Instructions

Heat oven to 400°.

Cook green beans around 5 minutes. Prepare beef meatballs as in the recipe above. Combine soup, flour, salt and pepper in a saucepan, stirring with a whisk until smooth. Bring to a boil over medium-high heat; cook 1 minute, stirring constantly. Remove from heat. Add yogurt dressing, beaten egg and then half of the cheese, stirring until well combined. Add sauce to green beans mixture; and stir gently until combined.
Put mixture in a small casserole dish oiled with some coconut oil. Sprinkle with remaining cheese. Bake at 400° for 50 minutes or until mixture bubbles at the edges and cheese begins to brown. Remove from oven and let cool for 5 minutes. Serve with large Fiber Loaded Salad with Italian Dressing.

"Breaded" "fried" food
Breaded Tilapia

Ingredients - Allergies: SF, GF, DF, NF

- 1/2 cup coconut meal for breading
- 1/4 tsp. pepper
- 1/4 tsp. minced garlic
- 1/4 tsp. paprika
- 1/8 tsp. salt
- 1 large egg whites (or whole eggs), beaten
- 1/2 pound tilapia fillets, cut into 1/2-by-3-inch strips

Instructions

Heat oven to 400°F. Set a wire rack on a baking sheet and coat with some coconut oil.

Place coconut, pepper, garlic, paprika and salt in a blender and process until finely ground. Transfer to a shallow dish.

Place egg whites in a second dish. Dip every piece of fish in the egg and then coat all sides with the coconut breading mixture. Place on the prepared rack. Sprinkle some drops of olive oil over each piece.

Bake until the fish is cooked through. Breading should be golden brown. Serve with large Fiber loaded salad.

Breaded Chicken

Ingredients - Allergies: SF, GF, DF, NF

- 1/2 cup flax seeds meal for breading
- 1/4 tsp. pepper
- 1/4 tsp. minced garlic
- 1/4 tsp. paprika
- 1/8 tsp. salt
- 1 large egg whites (or whole eggs), beaten
- 1/2 pound skinless, boneless chicken pieces

Instructions

Heat oven to 400°F. Set a wire rack on a baking sheet; coat with some coconut oil.

Place flax, pepper, garlic, paprika and salt in a food processor or blender and process until finely ground. Transfer to a shallow dish.

Place egg whites in a second dish. Dip every piece of chicken in the egg and then coat all sides with the flax breading mixture. Place on the prepared rack. Sprinkle some drops of olive oil over each piece.

Bake until the chicken is cooked through and the breading is golden brown and crisp, about 8 minutes each side. Serve with large Fiber loaded salad.

Lemon Pork with Asparagus

Ingredients - Allergies: SF, GF, DF, EF, NF

- 1/2 lb. pork chops
- 2 Tbsp. buckwheat flour
- 1/4 tsp. salt
- 1 tbsp. coconut oil
- Pepper
- 1/2 cup chopped asparagus
- 1 lemons, sliced

Instructions

Place the flour and salt in a dish and gently toss each chop in the dish to coat. Melt the coconut oil in a large skillet over medium high heat. Add the chicken and sauté until golden brown on each side. Sprinkle each side with the pepper directly in the pan.

When the chops are cooked through, transfer them to a plate. Add the lemon slices and asparagus to the pan. When the asparagus and the lemons are done, add the chops back to the pan.

Pizza

Meat Pizza

Ingredients - Allergies: SF, GF, EF, NF

- 1/2 cup cooked and minced chicken breast
- 1/2 cup low-fat cheddar, shredded
- 1/2 tbsp. minced onion & few basil leaves
- 1/2 tsp garlic minced

Instructions

Preheat oven to 425 degrees Fahrenheit. Process chicken, onion and garlic together. Mixture will be a dense crumb consistency. Press chicken mixture on parchment paper on a cookie sheet. Bake for 12 minutes. Let cool for five minutes.

Top with 1/4 cup of tomato sauce, a handful of low-fat cheese, basil and mushrooms (shiitake). Bake for 6-8 minutes more, or until toppings are melted. Let cool for five minutes. Slice and serve. Alternatively, you may want to try cauliflower crust version:

Grate half of the large cauliflower and steam it for 15 minutes. Squeeze the excess water out and let cool. Mix in 2 eggs, one cup low-fat mozzarella, and salt and pepper. Pat into a 10-inch round on the prepared cookie sheet. Brush with oil and bake until golden. Add the topping as above.

Crockpot

Slow Cooker Pepper Steak

Ingredients - Allergies: SF, GF, DF, EF, NF

- 1 pounds beef sirloin, cut into 2 inch strips
- 1/2 tbsp. minced garlic
- 1 tbsp. coconut oil
- 1/2 cup Beef Broth

- 1/2 tbsp. tapioca flour
- 1/4 cup chopped onion
- 1 cup carrots
- 1/2 cup chopped tomatoes
- 1/2 tsp. salt

Instructions

Sprinkle beef with minced garlic. Heat the coconut oil in a skillet and brown the seasoned beef sirloin strips. Transfer to a slow cooker.

Mix in tapioca flour in broth until dissolved. Pour broth into the slow cooker with meat. Add carrots, onion, chopped tomatoes and salt. Cover and cook on high for 3 to 4 hours, or on low for 6 to 8 hours.

Pork Tenderloin with peppers and onions

Ingredients - Allergies: SF, GF, DF, EF, NF

- 1 tbsp. coconut oil
- 3/4 pound pork loin
- 1/2 tbsp. caraway seeds
- 1/4 tsp sea salt
- 1/8 tsp ground black pepper
- 1/2 red onion, thinly sliced
- 1 red bell peppers, sliced
- 2 cloves of garlic, minced
- 1/4 cup chicken broth

Instructions

Wash and chop vegetables. Slice pork loin, and season with black pepper, caraway seeds and sea salt. Heat a pan over medium heat. Add coconut oil when hot. Add pork loin and brown slightly. Add onions and mushrooms, and continue to sauté until onions are translucent. Add peppers, garlic and chicken broth. Simmer until vegetables are tender and pork is fully cooked.

Beef Bourguinon

Ingredients - Allergies: SF, GF, DF, EF

- 3/4 or 1 pounds cubed lean beef
- 1/4 cup red wine
- 2 Tbsp. coconut oil
- 1/4 tsp. thyme
- 1/4 tsp. black pepper
- 1 cloves garlic, crushed
- 1/2 onion, diced
- 1/3 pound mushrooms, sliced
- 2 Tbsp. cup almond flour

Instructions

Marinate beef in wine, oil, thyme and pepper for few hours at room temperature or 6-8 hours in the fridge. Cook garlic and onion in a pan until soft. Add mushrooms. Cook until they are browned. Drain beef liquid. Place beef in slow cooker. Sprinkle flour over the beef and stir to coat. Add mushroom mixture on top. Pour reserved marinade over all. Cook on low for 7-9 hrs.

Italian Chicken

Ingredients - Allergies: SF, GF, DF, EF

- 2 pieces of skinless chicken
- 2 Tbsp. almond flour
- 1/2 tsp. salt
- 1/8 tsp. pepper
- 1/4 cup chicken broth
- 1/2 cup sliced mushrooms
- 1/4 tsp. paprika
- 1/2 zucchini, sliced into medium pieces
- ground black pepper
- parsley to garnish

Instructions

Season chicken with 1 tsp. salt. Combine flour, pepper, remaining salt, and paprika. Coat chicken pieces with this mixture. Place zucchini first in a crockpot. Pour broth over zucchini. Arrange chicken on top. Cover and cook on low for 6 to 8 hours or until tender. Turn control to high, add mushrooms, cover, and cook on high for additional 10-15 minutes. Garnish with parsley and ground black pepper.

Slow Cook Jambalaya

Ingredients - Allergies: SF, GF, DF, EF, NF

- 1/2 Bell pepper, chopped
- 1/2 Onion, chopped
- 1 Medium tomato, chopped
- 1/2 cup Chopped celery
- 1 Clove garlic, crushed
- 1 tbsp. minced parsley
- 1 tbsp. Chopped thyme leaves
- 1 tbsp. chopped Oregano leaves
- 1/8 tsp. Cayenne & 1/4 tsp. Salt
- 4 ounces pork, chopped
- 4 ounces Chicken breast, chopped
- 1 cups Beef broth
- 1/4 pound Cooked shelled shrimp
- 1/4 cup Cooked brown rice

Instructions

Shell shrimp and halve lengthwise. Combine all ingredients except shrimp & rice in a slow cooker. Cover & cook on low 9-10 hours. Turn slow cooker on high, add cooked shrimp & cooked rice. Cover; cook on high 20-30 minutes.

Ropa Vieja

Ingredients - Allergies: SF, GF, DF, EF, NF

- 1 tbsp. coconut oil
- 3/4 or 1 pound beef flank steak
- 1/2 cup beef broth
- 1/2 cup tomato sauce
- 1 small onion, sliced
- 1/2 green bell pepper sliced into strips
- 1 cloves garlic, chopped
- 1/4 cup tomato paste
- 1/2 tsp. ground cumin
- 1/2 tsp. chopped cilantro
- 1/2 tbsp. olive oil or avocado oil & 1 tbsp. lemon juice

Instructions

Heat oil in a skillet over high heat. Brown the flank steak on each side (4 minutes per side). Move the beef to a slow cooker. Add in the beef broth and tomato sauce, then add the onion, bell pepper, garlic , tomato paste , cumin, cilantro, olive oil and lemon juice. Stir until blended. Cover, and cook on high for 4 hours, or on Low for up to 8 hours. When ready to serve, shred meat and serve with salad.

Lemon Roast Chicken

Ingredients - Allergies: SF, GF, DF, EF, NF

- 2 pieces skinless chicken
- 1 dash Salt
- 1 dash Pepper
- 1 tsp. Oregano
- 1 cloves minced garlic
- 1 tbsp. coconut oil
- 1/4 cup Water
- 1 tbsp. Lemon juice

- Rosemary

Instructions

Wash chicken and season with salt and pepper. Sprinkle half of oregano and garlic inside chicken cavity. Add coconut oil to a frying pan. Brown chicken on all sides and transfer to crock pot. Sprinkle with oregano and garlic. Add water to fry pan and stir to loosen brown bits. Pour into crock pot and cover. Cook on low 7 hours. Add lemon juice when cooking is done. Transfer chicken to cutting board and carve chicken. Skim fat. Pour juice into sauce bowl. Serve with rosemary and some juice over chicken.

Fall Lamb and Vegetable Stew

Ingredients - Allergies: SF, GF, DF, EF, NF

- 3/4 or 1 pound Lamb stew meat
- 1 chopped Tomatoes
- 1/2 Summer squash
- 1/2 Zucchini
- 1/2 cup Mushrooms, sliced
- 1/2 cup Bell peppers, chopped
- 1/2 cup Onions, chopped
- 1/2 teaspoons Salt
- 1 Garlic cloves, crushed
- 1/4 tsp. Thyme leaves
- 1 Bay leaves
- 1 cups chicken broth

Instructions

Cut squash and zucchini. Place vegetables and lamb in crockpot. Mix salt, garlic, thyme, and bay leaf into broth and pour over lamb and vegetables. Cover and cook on low for 7 hours.

Slow cooker pork loin

Ingredients - Allergies: SF, GF, DF, EF, NF

- 3/4 pound of pork loin
- 1/2 cup tomato sauce
- 1 zucchinis, sliced
- 1/2 head cauliflower, separated into medium florets
- 1 Tbs dried basil
- 1/8 tsp ground black pepper
- 1/4 tsp sea salt (optional)

Instructions

Add all of the ingredients to a crock pot.

Cook on high for 3-4 hours or low 7-8 hours.

Sauerbraten

Ingredients - Allergies: SF, GF, DF, EF, NF

Marinade

- Water -- 1 cup
- Lemon juice – 1/4 cup
- Red wine – 1/2 cup
- Peppercorns – 1/2 tbsp.
- Juniper berries -- 4
- Whole cloves -- 2
- Bay leaves -- 1

Roast

- Beef rump or round -- 1 pound
- Salt and pepper -- to season
- coconut oil -- 1 tbsp.
- Onion, thinly sliced -- 1
- Carrot, cut into thin rounds -- 1
- Celery, thinly chopped -- 1 stalk

Instructions

Place the marinade ingredients (except lemon juice) into a pot and bring to a boil. Boil for 5 minutes then remove and cool to room temperature. Add lemon juice.

Place the beef in a large glass dish and pour the marinade. Make sure that beef is covered with the marinade.

Set the roast and its marinade in the fridge and marinade for at least few hours. Turn the beef once or twice daily.

Remove the roast from the marinade and season with salt and pepper. Brown the roast well on all sides and set aside.

Add the celery, onion and carrot to the pot and sauté until the onion is cooked translucent. Put the roast to the pot and add in the marinade. Bring to a boil, then reduce heat to medium-low. Cover the pot and simmer until the roast is fork tender.

Remove the roast and set it aside. Strain the sauce and discard the solids and return the liquid to the pot. Bring to a simmer and add in the salt and pepper and simmer for few minutes more.

Variations

- **Meats**: Pork, lamb or venison.
- **Marinade Variations**: Nutmeg, ginger, thyme and coriander.

Fish

Cioppino

Ingredients - Allergies: SF, GF, DF, EF, NF

- 1/4 cup coconut oil
- 1 onions, chopped
- 1 cloves garlic, minced
- 1/2 bunch fresh parsley, chopped
- 1/2 cup stewed tomatoes
- 1/2 cups chicken broth
- 1 bay leaves
- 1/2 tbsp. dried basil
- 1/4 tsp. dried thyme
- 1/4 tsp. dried oregano
- 1/2 cup water
- 1/2 cup white wine
- 1/2 pound peeled and deveined large shrimp
- 1/2 pound bay scallops
- 6 small clams
- 6 cleaned and debearded mussels
- 1/2 cups crabmeat
- 1/2 pounds cod fillets, cubed

Instructions

Over medium heat melt coconut oil in a large stockpot and add onions, parsley and garlic. Cook slowly, stirring occasionally until onions are soft. Add tomatoes to the pot. Add chicken broth, oregano, bay leaves, basil, thyme, water and wine. Mix well.

Cover and simmer 30 minutes.

Stir in the shrimp, scallops, clams, mussels and crabmeat. Stir in fish. Bring to boil. Lower heat, cover and simmer until clams open.

Flounder with Orange Coconut Oil

Ingredients - Allergies: SF, GF, DF, EF, NF

- 1 pound flounder
- 1 tbsp. white wine
- 1 tbsp. lemon juice
- 1 tbsp. coconut oil
- 1 tbsp. parsley
- 1/3 tsp. black pepper
- 1 tbsp. orange zest
- 1/4 tsp. salt
- 1/4 cup chopped scallions

Instructions

Preheat oven to 325F. Sprinkle fish with pepper and salt.
Place fish in the baking dish. Sprinkle orange zest on top of the fish. Melt remaining coconut oil and add the parsley and scallions to the coconut oil and pour over flounder. Then add in the white wine.
Place in oven and bake for 15 minutes. Serve fish with extra juice on a side.

Grilled Salmon

Ingredients - Allergies: SF, GF, DF, EF, NF

- 2 salmon filets
- 2 Tbsp. coconut oil
- 1 tbsp. fish sauce
- 1 tbsp. lemon juice
- 1 tbsp. thinly sliced green onion
- 1 clove garlic, minced & 1/4 tsp. ground ginger
- 1/4 tsp. crushed red pepper flakes
- 1/4 tsp. sesame oil
- 1/8 tsp. salt

Instructions

Whisk together coconut oil, fish sauce, garlic, ginger, red chili flakes, lemon juice, green onions, sesame oil, and salt. Put fish in a glass dish, and pour marinade over. Cover and refrigerate for 4 hours.
Preheat grill. Place salmon on grill. Grill until fish becomes tender. Turn halfway during cooking.

Crab Cakes

Ingredients - Allergies: SF, GF, DF, NF

- 1 lbs. crabmeat
- 1 beaten eggs
- 1 cup flax seeds meal
- 1 tbsp. mustard
- 1 tbsp. grated horseradish
- 1/4 cup coconut oil
- 1/2 tsp. lemon rind
- 1 tbsp. lemon juice
- 1 tbsp. parsley
- 1/4 tsp. cayenne pepper
- 1 tsp. fish sauce

Instructions

In medium bowl combine all ingredients except oil. Shape in to smallish hamburgers. In fry pan heat oil and cook patties for 3-4 minutes on each side or until golden brown. Optionally, bake them in the oven.
Serve as appetizers or as main course with large fiber salad.

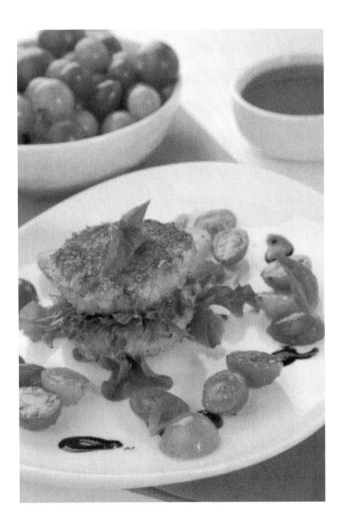

Sweets

Superfoods Dark Chocolate

Instructions - Allergies: SF, GF, DF, EF, V, NF

Mix 1/4 cup of coconut oil with 1/4 to 1/2 cup of cocoa powder (unsweetened, ideally organic and unprocessed) and some lucuma powder to taste. You really should experiment with cocoa and lucuma amount. Maybe start with equal amount of coconut oil, cocoa and lucuma, mix it and then increase amount of cocoa to your taste. Form balls or put in the ice cube tray. Put it in the fridge and 1 hour later you'll have great homemade Superfoods chocolate!

Fruits dipped in Superfoods chocolate

Ingredients - Allergies: SF, GF, DF, EF, V

- 1 apple or 1 banana or a bowl of strawberries or any fruit that can be dipped in melted chocolate
- 1/2 cup of melted superfoods chocolate (see earlier recipe)
- 2 tbsp. chopped nuts (almond, walnut, Brazil nuts) or seeds (hemp, chia, sesame, flax meal)

Instructions

Cut apple in wedges or cut banana in quarters. Melt the chocolate and chop the nuts. Dip fruit in chocolate, sprinkle with nuts or seeds and lay on tray. Transfer the tray to the fridge so the chocolate can harden; serve. If you don't want chocolate, cover fruits with almond or sunflower butter and sprinkle with chia or hemp seeds and cut it into chunks and serve.

Superfoods Ice cream

Allergies: SF, GF, DF, EF, V, NF

Freeze a banana cut into chunks and process it in blender once frozen and add half a tsp. of cinnamon or 1 tsp. of cocoa or both and eat it as ice-cream.

Other option would be to add one spoon of almond butter and mix it with mashed banana, it's also a delicious ice cream.

Whipped Coconut cream

Ingredients - Allergies: SF, GF, DF, EF, V, NF

- 2 cups of any fresh berries
- 1/2 lemons
- 1 can full fat coconut milk (14 oz.), refrigerated overnight
- 1 tsp of ground <u>vanilla</u> bean
- 2 Tbsp. lucuma powder
- Dash of cardamom, nutmeg and clove (optional)

Instructions

Separate coconut cream from the milk by putting it overnight in the fridge. Don't shake it before opening.

Open the can of coconut milk and scrape out the cream into a bowl. Use the saved milk for smoothies or other recipes.

Add cardamom, lucuma powder and vanilla. Whip the cream with a hand mixer until fluffy. Put in the fridge.

Wash berries and place in serving bowls or glasses. Squeeze the lemon over the berries. Place a big scoop of cream on top of the berries and serve.

Superfoods Reference Book

Unfortunately, I had to take out the whole Superfoods Reference Book out of all of my books because parts of that book are featured on my blog. I joined Kindle Direct Publishing Select program which allows me to have all my books free for 5 days every 3 months. Unfortunately, KDP Select program also means that all my books have to have unique content that is not available in any other online store or on the Internet (including my blog). I didn't want to remove parts of Superfoods Reference book that is already on my blog because I want that all people have free access to that information. I also wanted to be part of KDP Select program because that is an option to give my book for free to anyone. So, some sections of my Superfoods Reference Book can be found on my blog, under Superfoods menu on my blog. Complete Reference book is available for subscribers to my Superfoods Today Newsletter. Subscribers to my Newsletter will also get information whenever any of my books becomes free on Amazon. I will not offer any product pitches or anything similar to my subscribers, only Superfoods related information, recipes and weight loss and fitness tips. So, subscribe to my newsletter, download Superfoods Today Desserts free eBook which has complete Superfood Reference book included and have the opportunity to get all of my future books for free.

Your Free Gift

As a way of saying thanks for your purchase, I'm offering you my FREE eBook that is exclusive to my book and blog readers.

Superfoods Cookbook Book Two has over 70 Superfoods recipes and complements Superfoods Cookbook Book One and it contains Superfoods Salads, Superfoods Smoothies and Superfoods Deserts with ultra-healthy non-refined ingredients. All ingredients are 100% Superfoods.

It also contains Superfoods Reference book which is organized by Superfoods (more than 60 of them, with the list of their benefits), Superfoods spices, all vitamins, minerals and antioxidants. Superfoods Reference Book lists Superfoods that can help with 12 diseases and 9 types of cancer.

http://www.SuperfoodsToday.com/FREE

Other Books from this Author

Superfoods Today Diet is a Kindle Superfoods Diet <u>book</u> that gives you 4 week Superfoods Diet meal plan as well as 2 weeks maintenance meal plan and recipes for weight loss success. It is an extension of Detox book and it's written for people who want to switch to Superfoods lifestyle.

Superfoods Today Body Care is a Kindle <u>book</u> with over 50 Natural Recipes for beautiful skin and hair. It has body scrubs, facial masks and hair care recipes made with the best Superfoods like avocado honey, coconut, olive oil, oatmeal, yogurt, banana and Superfoods herbs like lavender, rosemary, mint, sage, hibiscus, rose.

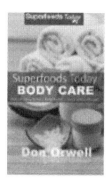

Superfoods Today Cookbook is a Kindle <u>book</u> that contains over 160 Superfoods recipes created with 100% Superfoods ingredients. Most of the meals can be prepared in under 30 minutes and some are really quick ones that can be done in 10 minutes only. Each recipe combines Superfoods ingredients that deliver astonishing amounts of antioxidants, essential fatty acids (like omega-3), minerals, vitamins, and more.

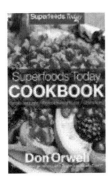

Superfoods Today Smoothies is a Kindle Superfoods Smoothies <u>book</u> with over 70+ 100% Superfoods smoothies. Featured are Red, Purple, Green and Yellow Smoothies

Low Carb Recipes for Diabetics is a Kindle Superfoods book with Low Carb Recipes for Diabetics.

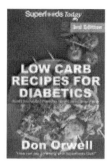

Diabetes Recipes is a Kindle Superfoods book with Superfoods Diabetes Recipes suitable for Diabetes Type-2.

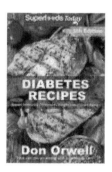

Diabetic Cookbook for One is a Kindle Superfoods <u>book</u> with Diabetes Recipes for One suitable for Diabetes Type-2

Diabetic Meal Plans is a Kindle <u>book</u> with Superfoods Diabetes Meal Plans suitable for Diabetes Type-2

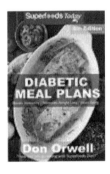

One Pot Cookbook is a Kindle Superfoods <u>book</u> with Superfoods One Pot Recipes.

Low Carb Dump Meals is a Kindle <u>book</u> with Low Carb Dump Meals Superfoods Recipes.

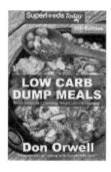

Superfoods Today Salads is a Kindle book that contains over 60 Superfoods Salads recipes created with 100% Superfoods ingredients. Most of the salads can be prepared in 10 minutes and most are measured for two. Each recipe combines Superfoods ingredients that deliver astonishing amounts of antioxidants, essential fatty acids (like omega-3), minerals, vitamins, and more.

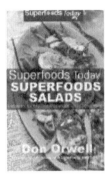

Superfoods Today Kettlebells is a Kindle Kettlebells beginner's book aimed at 30+ office workers who want to improve their health and build stronger body without fat.

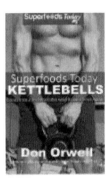

Superfoods Today Red Smoothies is a Kindle Superfoods Smoothies book with more than 40 Red Smoothies.

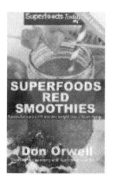

Superfoods Today 14 Days Detox is a Kindle Superfoods Detox book that gives you 2 week Superfoods Detox meal plan and recipes for Detox success.

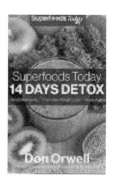

Superfoods Today Yellow Smoothies is a Kindle Superfoods Smoothies book with more than 40 Yellow Smoothies.

Superfoods Today Green Smoothies is a Kindle Superfoods Smoothies book with more than 35 Green Smoothies.

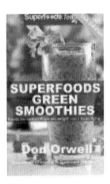

Superfoods Today Purple Smoothies is a Kindle Superfoods Smoothies book with more than 40 Purple Smoothies.

Superfoods Cooking For Two is a Kindle book that contains over 150 Superfoods recipes for two created with 100% Superfoods ingredients.

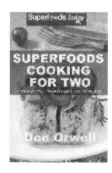

Nighttime Eater is a Kindle <u>book</u> that deals with Nighttime Eating Syndrome (NES). Don Orwell is a life-long Nighttime Eater that has lost his weight with Superfoods and engineered a solution around Nighttime Eating problem. Don still eats at night☺. Don't fight your nature, you can continue to eat at night, be binge free and maintain low weight.

Superfoods Today Smart Carbs 20 Days Detox is a Kindle Superfoods <u>book</u> that will teach you how to detox your body and start losing weight with Smart Carbs. The book has over 470+ pages with over 160+ 100% Superfoods recipes.

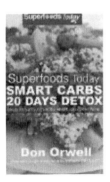

Superfoods Today Vegetarian Salads is a Kindle book that contains over 40 Superfoods Vegetarian Salads recipes created with 100% Superfoods ingredients. Most of the salads can be prepared in 10 minutes and most are measured for two.

Superfoods Today Vegan Salads is a Kindle book that contains over 30 Superfoods Vegan Salads recipes created with 100% Superfoods ingredients. Most of the salads can be prepared in 10 minutes and most are measured for two.

Superfoods Today Soups & Stews is a Kindle <u>book</u> that contains over 70 Superfoods Soups and Stews recipes created with 100% Superfoods ingredients.

Superfoods Desserts is a Kindle Superfoods Desserts <u>book</u> with more than 60 Superfoods Recipes.

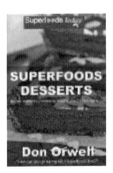

Smoothies for Diabetics is a Kindle <u>book</u> that contains over 70 Superfoods Smoothies adjusted for diabetics.

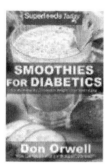

50 Shades of Superfoods for Two is a Kindle <u>book</u> that contains over 150 Superfoods recipes for two created with 100% Superfoods ingredients.

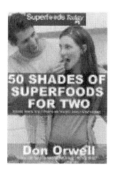

50 Shades of Smoothies is a Kindle book that contains over 70 Superfoods Smoothies.

50 Shades of Superfoods Salads is a Kindle book that contains over 60 Superfoods Salads recipes created with 100% Superfoods ingredients. Most of the salads can be prepared in 10 minutes and most are measured for two. Each recipe combines Superfoods ingredients that deliver astonishing amounts of antioxidants, essential fatty acids (like omega-3), minerals, vitamins, and more.

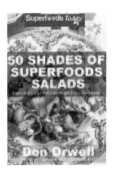

Superfoods Vegan Desserts is a Kindle Vegan Dessert <u>book</u> with 100% Vegan Superfoods Recipes.

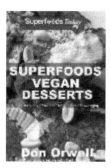

Desserts for Two is a Kindle Superfoods Desserts <u>book</u> with more than 40 Superfoods Desserts Recipes for two.

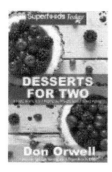

Superfoods Paleo Cookbook is a Kindle Paleo <u>book</u> with more than 150 100% Superfoods Paleo Recipes.

Superfoods Breakfasts is a Kindle Superfoods <u>book</u> with more than 40 100% Superfoods Breakfasts Recipes.

Superfoods Dump Dinners is a Kindle Superfoods <u>book</u> with Superfoods Dump Dinners Recipes.

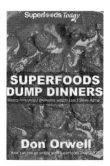

Healthy Desserts is a Kindle Desserts <u>book</u> with more than 50 100% Superfoods Healthy Desserts Recipes.

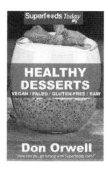

Superfoods Salads in a Jar is a Kindle Salads in a Jar <u>book</u> with more than 35 100% Superfoods Salads Recipes.

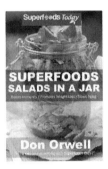

Smoothies for Kids is a Kindle Smoothies <u>book</u> with more than 80 100% Superfoods Smoothies for Kids Recipes.

Vegan Cookbook for Beginners is a Kindle Vegan <u>book</u> with more than 75 100% Superfoods Vegan Recipes.

Vegetarian Cooking for Beginners is a Kindle Vegetarian <u>book</u> with more than 150 100% Superfoods Paleo Recipes.

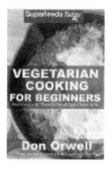

Foods for Diabetics is a Kindle <u>book</u> with more than 170 100% Superfoods Diabetics Recipes.

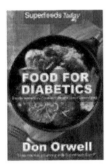

Healthy Kids Cookbook is a Kindle <u>book</u> with Superfoods Kids friendly Recipes.

Superfoods Beans Recipes is a Kindle <u>book</u> with Superfoods Beans Recipes.

Diabetic Slow Cooker Recipes is a Kindle <u>book</u> with Superfoods Slow Cooker Diabetic Recipes.

Ketogenic Crockpot Recipes is a Kindle <u>book</u> with Superfoods Ketogenic Crockpot Recipes.

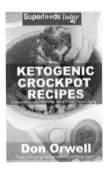

Stir Fry Cooking is a Kindle <u>book</u> with Stir Fry Superfoods Recipes.

Sirt Food Diet Cookbook is a Kindle <u>book</u> with Superfoods Sirt Food Recipes.

Printed in Great Britain
by Amazon